This book is intended as a reference volume only, not as a medical text. The information provided herein is designed to help you make informed decisions about your health. It is not intended to be a substitute for any treatment that may have been prescribed by your doctor. It is sold with the understanding that the publisher is not engaged in rendering medical advice. If you have a medical problem, we urge you to seek competent medical help.

HT Press LLC

Copyright © 2014 Zatiti Ema, MA
First published in 2015 by

HT Press
Montgomery Village, MD 20886

Sh. SAungkt Akhu Nnebu.
Makini Niliwaambieni,
Sheeba Ema-Nuru

Cover Artist: Mshindo Kuumba

Electronic page layout: Charles Lowder   charleslowder@verizon.net

Although the author and publisher have made every effort to ensure that the information in this book was correct at press time, the author and publisher do not assume and hereby disclaim any liability to any party for any loss, damage, or disruption caused by errors or omissions, whether such errors or omissions result from negligence, accident, or any other cause. Including links we have provided.

TXu001906180 / 2014-02-11

Ema, Zatiti. MA
    Our Journey: Red, Black, Green and Vegan.

ISBN 978-1-4951-3341-1

Library of Congress Control Number: 2015920629

OUR JOURNEY

RED, BLACK, GREEN

AND

VEGAN

Zatiti Ema, MA

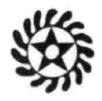

DEDICATION

I would like to first acknowledge the Creator Father-Mother God or giving me this incredible life and life force which has directed me to live on a higher consciousness, of which eating from the plant kingdom is a part. I would like to acknowledge my personal and communal ancestors, angels and guides who work with me in mysterious ways.

I humbly dedicate this book to the tireless health warriors, queens and African freedom fighters who have worked to uplift the African community through health education. Some of the noted include the staff at the Institute of Positive Education, Third World Press, Phil Kelan Cohran, Dr. Alvenia Fulton (RIP), Dick Gregory, Queen Afua, Dr. Africa, Ra Un Nefer Amen and the Ausar Auset Society, the Honorable Elijah Muhammad (RIP), Aris Latham, Swami Krishnapada (RIP), Hebrew Israelites Nation, the Rastafarian community, Dr. Sebi and the new kids on the block, Dr. Enki, and Dr Ali Muhammad.

A special dedication to the man who gave his seed and his life lessons so that I might see; my father and my mother who taught me that healthy living wasn't for everybody. May you both rest in power. To my kind, and most of the time vegan daughter, Sheeba Ema Nuru, Rick Wright for pushing me to write and my sistah friend Dr. Alyce Sherman, for her wonderful support in getting this project rolling.

I would also like to thank the following who contributed recipes or their thoughts:

Mark Blake

Linda Carter

Elaine Rice-Fells

Chef Heru aka Harold Goodridge

Dr. Akua Gray

Kunti Hawkins

Tomi Makanjuola

Dr. Baruch Ben-Yehudah

Rasafik Weusi

Table of Contents

✳ Ananse Ntontan

✵ Nsoromma

FOREWORD

When the love for self is so great it drives you to do without excuses what is good for the body, mind and spirit.

Being young, gifted, and intelligent means nothing if you are not well. Therefore, the lifestyle of wellness that begins when you're young can only have dynamic results for the one who takes care of themselves at an early age. Imagine never being sick a day in your life. Imagine having the stamina and strength to fulfill every task physical, mental or spiritual that comes your way for your personal growth and progress. YOU CAN DO IT!

It begins with a commitment to loving and caring for yourself despite what others are doing around you. Be PHAT! Be CUT! Be all that! When you put in the work, you deserve it!

Zatiti Ema shows you the 1 - 2 - 3's of living life and living life well! This easy to follow guide is a timeless tool for the youth and young adults to accelerate in their health goals to master father time and align themselves with Mother Nature!

Sending Light to All That You Make Beautiful in the World,
Dr. Akua

INTRODUCTION

I wrote this book as I grew weary of answering questions in relation to how to be or become a plant eater. Questions on how to stay healthy. Questions about how I kept my weight down. I wanted to develop an easy read that would appeal to the average soul in the Nubian world (so-called Black, herein also referenced as African).

Time will only tell if I have met my objectives. I wanted my readers to know of the Nubian/African organizations in the community that advocated for healthy cuisine as one of the tools toward liberation in diaspora. So I wrote this book with much help and support from my sistah editors including Dr. Alyce Sherman, Sheeba Ema-Nuru, Makini Niliwaambieni, Sh. SAungkt Akhu Nnebu.

The colors Red, Black & Green, were taken from the teachings of the Honorable Marcus Garvey and Dr. Malichi Z. York. They both used the colors to stand for the liberation of all African People. The colors represent freedom to many. They represent liberation from global European oppression. But we have expanded the meaning to include Freedom from eating the dead and the foods of the dead. The Adinkra symbols pictured at the beginning of each section are apart of West African culture gifted to the world through the Ashanti People of Ghana.

In this book you will learn how I turned to a plant-based diet. I will show the you what foods to avoid. I will give you steps to begin your journey to eating, shopping and knowing more about what's going into your body temple.

You will learn that it's not just about food-- there are many variables including water, supplements, and the types of containers you prepare your food in. The reader will be exposed to many ideas in the plant based diet. This book can be used as a reference tool in your healing kitchen. Health really begins there, not in a fast food joint or in the gas station. I've written a book full of charts and lists so in your busy lives you can get the information in a glance. I have included many starter recipes, both my own and the work of others. This book is not meant to be a cook book or even a non-cook book (living/raw food). It is meant to help you make the transition to a healthy lifestyle. The recipes are just a bonus to get you started.

You will learn that you can take baby steps or giant steps on your healing journey. Whatever you decide to do, know that eating flesh is old school. It is old school as it inflicts cruelty upon animals. It is old school as it is not in the best interest of the human body to consume dead animals. It is old school as it is not sustainable for our beautiful planet. It wastes gasoline, electricity, food and the animal feces pollute our waterways. It is old school as the animals eat plants for their needs. We can do the same.

I hope after reading my offering, you understand that this is not an all or nothing game. You can choose. You can choose to eat plants, one day a week or seven. You can choose to eat a plant based diet one meal a day or all three. You choose, it is your planet and your body temple. It is your karma. Do your best and pray for strength along the way. You will have many tools to help you. Fight apathy which will emerge as you take this journey. Fight it with a plan. Plan what you are going to eat the next day before the sun sets. This will help you more than you realize.

The choice is yours. Do your best and go forward with prayer, affirmations and visualization. Welcome to the Journey to Red, Black, Green and Vegan.

Sankofa

Better Late than Never

In The Beginning

I was raised in the Northwest by young, southern parents, who in an effort to escape the racism of the south, migrated to Portland, Oregon in 1953 with three children in tow. Little did they know—racism was not just particular to the south.

My grandfather Elijah, who was already living in Portland with his wife, had purchased a home in the northeast section of the city and encouraged my parents to join them. Many African-Americans took part in this migration to the northwest, as cheap labor was needed for the building of ships during World War II. My family travelled by train to Oregon and moved in with my grandfather and his second wife Ruth. *(I would learn later in life that Ruth left my grandfather to join a Hebrew Israelite group, who are plant eaters as well).*

The house seemed massive to me. Perched on a hill with a large porch for family gatherings, it had many stairs within its two stories and a basement. I can recall many days of playing hide-and-go-seek with my brothers. The house became an indoor playground for us. Daddy Elijah's wife was not too happy to have all of that robust energy in her otherwise elegant home. My father soon got a job at a meat packing plant in North Portland, refusing to work the shipyards. We later moved to our own home in Southeast Portland and began a new chapter in life.

When I was 16, my father taught me how to drive and I would often keep his car during the day and pick him up from work at the end of his shift. This is how I got my first glimpse of what went on at the meat packing plant. We called it the slaughterhouse at home, but when dad spoke to someone important he would say meat packing plant.

One afternoon, I arrived at my father's job early. I grew tired of waiting in the hot car so I got out in my spring cottons and nice shoes *(that I thought were so cute)*. I remember worrying about my shoes getting dusty as they touched the gravel and dirt as I walked. I began strolling toward what would become for me an unbelievably hellish scene. The outer portion of the facility did not face the street but was off a main road, over the railroad tracks, and down a block before you even reached the parking lot. It was as if the owners did not want the world to be witness to the slaughterhouse and its animal horrors.

I was not prepared for what I was about to see. Animals were being herded into a line and appeared to be in distress as if they knew what was about to happen to them.

A large hook came down from a conveyor belt and grab the animal under the chin bone, mandible, and the still-alive animal was lifted into the air and herded hanging on the conveyor belt into the packing house facility. The animal was then cut open down the anterior and its organs fell to the cement floor with a dreadful splat. Blood was everywhere! I stood in shock. Traumatized by this brutality.

My father, outfitted in a rubber suit and boots was standing nearby with a broom and water hose sweeping up the bloody mess. When my father, visually anguished by my presence, told me to leave- he did not have to tell me twice.

Sankofa

I was nauseated by what I was witnessing. On what had moments before been for me a beautiful, sunny afternoon, a day on which I had looked forward to spending one on one time with my Baba, was suddenly gone. Now none of that mattered. I was shocked and saddened for the animals who lost their lives in such a cold and cruel way and for my father who had to work in such a hideous environment. I went back to the parking lot in a dazed and depressed state, but not before noting that when they finished slaughtering one species of animals they would clean the area and start with the next. First cows and then pigs. It was sensory overload for me — I never wanted to go inside the slaughterhouse again in life.

When I am in the supermarket, my spirit becomes uneasy as I walk pass the sections in which the butcher prepares the carcass of the dead animal beings for human consumption. I always wonder why the smell and the extreme coldness of refrigeration does not alert other humans to, what is in my opinion, the tragedy associated with the consumption of dead animals. I feel blessed to have been gifted with a consciousness in this regard.

I encouraged my father to seek a different position or return to school. His response was "with three kids and a wife to care for, pursuing my education is not going to happen". He lacked any optimism. And that...was that.

He continued working in the slaughterhouse. The pressures of keeping our family financially stable and going to his blood-drenched job everyday was too much for my father and he eventually turned to alcohol to dull the pains of life. If only he had turned to meditation/prayer.

His work environment was also full of racism. He became the recipient of degrading racial slurs and insults, to which he remained silent, but anger welled inside of him. When intoxicated, my father displayed his most hideous lower self that was cold, mean, and sometimes cruel. I assume the slaughterhouse taught him to be insensitive to cruelty. A lesson he unfortunately learned too well. When sober, he was fatherly, humorous, attentive, supportive and caring. A Dr. Jekyll and Mr. Hyde as it were. Did he become a product of his environment?

During this period, I was desensitized by the euphemisms commonly used for dead animal flesh. Dead animal flesh is never called what it truly is, but is referred to as beef, steak, patties, hamburger, bacon and other labels. I, like most people, had no idea as to the degree of inhumanity that went into the meat processing industry. We only saw the neatly packaged meat in the store and did not connect our breakfast and dinner with the violence and suffering of these dead animals. I did not realize that I was advocating this process every time I ate a meal of dead animal flesh. The experience at the meat packing plant did not immediately bring me to a plant based diet. I logged the experience as disturbing, yet I went along with the program of eating dead animals everywhere I went – school, church, restaurants – with family, and friends. At the age of 16, I did not know that there was another way. Nor did I have the strength to buck the family traditions.

There was one other incident which I recall. This occurred in our southeast Portland, single-family, bungalow home. My father purchased a side of beef from his job at a very good price. He saved money because he and my mother would have to complete the butchering and preparation of the animal for consumption by our family. My father and brothers carried the carcass of the cow into our basement. My father had the basement sanitized and prepared as if in preparation for an event. The children were then told to go upstairs as my father realized that the job of cutting up 100 plus pounds of a cow's flesh would be a most unpleasant image for his children.

We went upstairs as instructed by our parents but curiosity got the best of us. We ever so silently crept down the basement steps, down the long hall with cold cement under our brown feet, past the wood stove and peeked into the basement utility room. There we saw our parents, covered in blood and wielding knives, dissecting the flesh of this seemingly huge animal. I was instantly sickened and struck with grief and remorse to see our parents participating in such a hideous process. It was particularly upsetting to see my beautiful, petite, freckled faced mother covered in blood. They saw us standing at the door of what had been transformed into a basement slaughterhouse with horrified looks on our faces. They yelled at us to go back upstairs. We ran down the hall and up the stairs not wanting to return—ever. We were later called to help clean up with brooms, mops and a water hose. The heavy scent of blood was everywhere and loomed in my mind as a morbid memory.

I did not realize then that these events would later shape my adult life and help transform me into a person who only consumes for the most part plants, seeds, nuts, herbs, greens, grains, sprouts, and fruits.

When I transgress from this main diet, I do not beat myself up. Nor do I allow myself to get away with murder, and go off the deep end with items that are processed or not for my highest good.

Balance is key in making choices about anyTHANG!

Time passed and I decided to attend the University of Oregon where I ate pretty much what the other students ate... too much starch, sweets-sugar, salt, dead animals, overcooked vegetables, and processed chemicals posing as junk food. I can remember going to McDonald's and ordering a Big Mac and fries. I did however take note of Elijah Muhammad's books and the Muslim teachings on the pig as well as some vegetables and realized that we should not eat just everything. I went to graduate school in Michigan at the age of 21. I enrolled in the Urban Counseling program. Many students were politically conscious, aware of vegetarianism, and practicing on a variety of levels. By this time I had stopped eating pork and was cutting back on red bloody meat.

One of my roommates was an African sistah from Liberia who did not like the way I prepared food. She was unaccustomed to eating large portions of meat with only a little vegetables and white potatoes. She informed me of how unhealthy my cooking regimen was and we agreed that I would keep the home clean and she would cook. I immediately noticed that she prepared meals as stews/soups, with less meat and more vegetable in a tasty sauce with rice or some other grain. Meat was still on the plate, just not in the quantity I was used to eating.

I really enjoyed my roommate's cooking and made a concerted effort to learn from her. Most of our meals were a combination of vegetables, chicken or fish, and her vegetables were simply delicious. I have fond memories of her collard greens cooked in coconut milk. We would frequently have plantains and everything always had wonderful flavors and aromas.

She had a practice of always leaving a little saucer of food for her ancestors in the kitchen. My roommate did not tell me initially that the saucers of food were for the ancestors and I would eat the food. When she shared the purpose of the food with me I felt silly for what I had done but soon began to understand that every day we ate, the ancestors also eat and were remembered.

I continued to read Elijah Muhammad's book *How to Eat to Live* and also picked up a book entitled *Back to Eden* that would become my constant companion as a resource in my kitchen. I noted that the author Jethro Kloss went even further than Elijah Muhammad with the belief that eating dead pigs was not a wise health practice. They both emphasized that we should not eat anything that moves. I was amazed with this theory/concept that humans did not need flesh foods. His book also motivated me to investigate the notion of using herbs as a method to heal oneself. I later learned from my mom that my great grandmother in Arkansas was a well-known and respected self-taught herbalist who worked with a Native Medicine man in her home town to keep the African people well. So when I became intrigued with health and aspects of healing, my mother was not surprised. They felt as if I was following in the line of my ancestors and elders came to me for consultations about their health when I visited.

While attending a lecture by Dr. Haki Madhubuti at Michigan State University where he spoke about the liberation of African (Nubian) People in America, African culture and returning our people to our African identity using those traditions, as a method to heal our community. I was so impressed and moved by his consciousness that I moved to Chicago to work with his grassroots Pan African organization at the time called IPE, the Institute of Positive Education. We were on the vanguard of many fronts, including plant-based diets.

Our desire, individual and collective, was to help our people release the shackles of Westernization and reinvent the African mind, family, and community in the West. Women were respected as leaders and valued for their daily professional tasks as well as cooking, nurturing, and educating the children. They spoke freely without restriction or domination by their male counterparts—very different from what I had witnessed in other communities.

In Chicago, working with Dr. Haki and the other brothers and sisters in the movement, I noted that this group of Black intellectuals was "def jam" on their diet. They did not play with their palette. They juiced, took supplements, and they did not eat meat. Most of the individuals I encountered through Third World Press and the Institute of Positive Education were older than I. I thought perhaps they were just extremists with their diets and I did not intend on joining them.

One of the practices of this African intellectual community, was a morning run. I was about 23 years old and this was right up my alley. We met at the park between 6 am and 7 am several mornings and began doing our warm-ups and laps around the perimeter of the park on Ellis Street. Most lived in that same community so this made doing things together easy. The brothers and sisters who were running were generally 10 years older, yet I could not keep up with them. I remember them passing me as I coughed and spat up the excess mucus released by my body. They lovingly teased me about my diet as they each passed me by.

I now had to take a serious step towards learning and later incorporating this knowledge into my active lifestyle.

Mama Johari Amini, a practicing nutritionist/dietician, University professor and founding member of IPE, taught me how to juice and directed me toward books on therapeutic juicing. She would juice after our run as she prepared to sit at her desk and work. One spring morning I saw her juice a cucumbers and drink it, I was in shock! At the time, she was married to speaker/author Jawanza Kunjufu who was also a plant eater. Although she was older than her husband, it was not evident upon sight, most likely due in part to her diet and lifestyle. These heavy African/Nubian thinkers and doers did not drink or smoke. Doing drugs was not even a remote consideration. I somehow felt that the diet also helped these people to be the intellectual/artist & revolutionaries that they were.

Mama Safisha Madhubuti, (Dr. Carol Lee), Haki's wife, would take me out for a vegetarian or vegan dinner and continue teaching me the path of a plant eater.

Our lifestyle was vastly different from many around us in the 70s. IPE held classes to help people make the transition from a devitalized flesh diet to a plant-based diet.

I also had the opportunity to work/study with 'Kelan' Phil Cohran, founding member of the AACM, (the Association for the Advancement of Creative Musicians) a vegan health educator, musician, composer, and astrologer. He held classes in his south side Chicago studio. Many of his classes were devoted to cooking vegetarian meals. Another health pioneer in Chicago, whom I knew as Dr. Fulton, had a fantastic herb and health food store. She led me to the works of Dick Gregory who was one of her students and an advocate of plant-based diet and fasting. Dr. Fulton taught Mr. Gregory how to fast and I also became one of her students as she taught me how to properly fast as well. She placed me on a 40-day supervised fast in which I became clairvoyant for a period. Amazing!

This entire experience along with my introduction to the African Hebrew Israelites, another group existing entirely on a non-meat diet, was life changing. Black African Chicago was a thriving pyramid with African Natural Health practitioners, health food stores, juice bars, and natural food restaurants to feed the desires of the wholistic food movement of the time period. It was wonderful to live during this time and be a open to new ideas.

While living in Chicago, I was also exposed to the teachings of a people who called themselves the devotees of Lord Krishna. They had a large African following, including my roommate Kadi. They also advocated a plant based diet. They however included dairy products in their diet as they believed the cow was sacred and so was its milk.

When I had the opportunity to travel to the beautiful lush island of Jamaica, I met many brothers and sistahs who were vegetarian/vegans and Rastafarians. I later moved to Africa and my roommate at that time was a Rasta, and a dancer with the famous drummer Olatunji, may he rest in peace. Olabisi was a plant eater from whom I learned much. Knowledge of the vegetarian/vegan diet has been in the African American community for some time and advocated by many different groups. Now many Nubian Christian fellowships are awakening to the benefits of a diet free from dead animal flesh and the five whites.

I later moved to Missouri to Unity Village to study metaphysics and work in the silent unity prayer room. Although they were supporters of a plant based diet, they would accommodate meat eaters in their public areas. I was impressed to find that the cafeteria at the village had an entire section for plant eaters. I was most happy when in environments that honored this aspect of my lifestyle.

Sankofa

While in Missouri, I became a radio and cable television producer/host. This gave me the opportunity to expose even more people to ideas on eating from the earth. My daughter was born during this period. During her first three years she grew on mother's milk and then almond and sesame seed milk before moving on to fruits and grains. I did not know about sprouted grains at the time. I followed the teaching of the African Hebrew Israelites and the Seventh Day Adventists on how to raise a veggie baby.

At one point I took my daughter to a restaurant and was overwhelmed by the scent of fish and ordered fish--a rare occurrence. My daughter perhaps 4 years old said to me, "What is that?" I played it off, "Oh it's fish--not as bad for us as meat." She said, "Mom we don't eat dead animals." I responded, "Yea it's ok--once in a great while." She said, "Mom it has eyes and it moves, we don't eat animals!" Then she asked, "Does it have a mom?" She was surprisingly determined to stop this transgression!

Transitioning

While working in the District of Columbia, I developed a nasty ear infection. I can recall a yellow-green   material draining out of my ear. This was during the period that I was terribly addicted to cheese. I remember having frequent head colds but I did not let these short episodes derail me from my love affair with cow's milk cheese. I understood that many people of African descent are lactose intolerant but I continued eating my beloved toxic cheese. When I came down with the ear infection, I knew beyond a shadow of a doubt that it was the writing on the wall. I called one of my favorite medically trained naturopaths, Dr. Gerald Douglas. Dr. Douglas was trained in Portland, Oregon at the College of Natural Medicine, which gave us a special connection. I remember calling him from my apartment outside of the District to get his recommendation regarding the challenges I was experiencing.

I sat on the floor in the hallway as he gave me his recommendation. He told me in a no-holds barred tone to get myself to the emergency room, take the drugs they prescribed and that he could not do anything more for me until that infection was cleared out. As a naturalist, I did not want to go to the hospital nor take any drugs. I do not like putting unnatural substances in my body. Dr. Douglas' advice shook me up and made me realize if I was going to be healthy and stay out of western medical institutions, I would need to grow up and stop eating low frequency foods like dairy.

I followed his instructions to go to the emergency room and take the prescribed drugs. I quit stuffing my face with animal cheese...well, for the most part. I still like cheese, but now I realize how damaging this addiction can be to my body temple so I began buying vegan cheese made from rice milk instead. I also learned not to eat it regularly. This gives the temple a rest and a period of detoxification. Vegan cheese is not as tasty as cow's cheese, so have your spices ready. See Linda Carter's raw vegan cheese creation in the raw recipe section. Cow's milk cheese can be a very real addiction. Visiting websites such as www.notmilk.com can be illuminating and offers encouragement to kick it.

These experiences all contributed to my final transformation to a vegetarian, then a vegan. As I continued to grow and study, I was introduced to a raw plant-based diet by my then good friend and health advocate, Nandini Devi Dasi aka Beverly Towns—peace be upon her soul—who owned Fountains of Life in Washington D. C. Together we attended classes and studied with premier raw foodist, Aris Latham. I continued my studies at the Ann Wigmore Institute of Living Foods Lifestyle. While struggling with brain trauma from a car collision, and later gallstones partly due to not drinking enough water, my healing was accelerated when I moved to a 80% living/raw diet and supplementation.

I have worked with and supported raw food chef, author, and owner of Khepra Raw Food and Juice bar Khepra Anu with many of his fasting detox projects. I run a Detox Day Spa with numerous modalities to clean out the body as well as Wholistic Health Consultant and mobile massage business. I frequently teach classes, workshops, and serve as a lecturer for groups and organizations on a variety of topics.

This is my sojourn into dining primarily with plants. My journey from a Southern/slave diet, to a S.A.D. (Standard American Diet), to a palate of vegetarian/vegan foods that have and give life— perhaps the diet of ascension. I know that my offering will help you with your growth and development toward conscious eating.

My journey has revealed that the universe demands that we grow or we are destined to repeat lessons until we awaken and take the higher, less popular paths. I encourage you to make a shift in your eating and see what gear you land in. I am sure you will be grateful and pleased. As you keep shifting you will certainly continue to advance your souls script.

May the beings of light, love, and compassion have their way on our planet and in the multi-verse.

The journey of healing is seemingly infinite. I wish you the highest and the best!

Nubian/African/Black
Vegans, Vegetarians & Live Foodists

Dr. Llaila Afrika
Queen Afua
Dr. Sunyatta Amen
Khepra Anu
India Arie
Erykah Badu
Angela Bassett
Andre "3000" Benjamin
Free "Akua" Benjamin
Beyonce
Chef Linda Carter
Phil Cohran
Zak Condo
Ur Aua Hehimetu Ra
  Enkamit
Omar Epps
Dr. Akua Gray
Ayana Gregory
Dick Gregory
C. Heru/Harold
  Goodridge
Dr. & Mrs. Hawkins
Tom Joyner
Coretta Scott King
Mshindo Kummba
Dr. Jawanza Kunjufu
Carl Lewis
Dr. George Love

Abut Maat
Dr. Haki R. Madhubuti
Taj Mahal
Shavonne Morton
Johnny Nash
Ra Un Nefer
Sheeba Ema Nuru
Swami Krishna Pad
Rosa Parks
Prince
Felicia Rashad
Elaine Rice-Fells
Ruben Stoddard
Shekhem Tepraim Saa
Cicely Tyson
Mike Tyson
Dr. Phil Valentine
Forrest Whitaker
Dr. Baruch Ben Yehda
Zakhah

*The most vegans reside in
the US, England and India.
Less than1% of the
Americans are vegans

Nyansapo

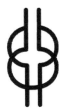

Wisdom and Integrity

Why Eat A Plant-Based Diet?

I f you are interested in historical traditions tied to the non-consumption of animals this next section is sure to interest you. If history is not your thang, skip this section.

Here are some ancient Kamitan sources which indicate that certain animals were not consumed. It also gives reference to cleansing and purification.

The first one is from the **Coffin Text 157** from Kamit:

"...O Batit of the evening, you swamp-dwellers, you of Mendes, ye of Buto, you of the shade of Ra which knows not praise, you who brew stoppered beer---do you know why Rekhyt [Lower Egypt] was given to He-ru? It was Ra who gave it to him in recompense for the injury in his eye. It was Ra--he said to Heru: "Pray, let me see your eye since this has happened to it" [injured in the fight with Set]. Then Ra saw it. Ra said: "Pray, look at that injury in your eye, while your hand is a covering over the good eye which is there." Then Heru looked at that injury. It assumed the form of a black pig. Thereupon Heru shrieked because of the state of his eye, which was stormy [inflamed]. Heru said: "Behold, my eye is as at that first blow which Set made against my eye!" Thereupon Heru swallowed his heart before him [lost consciousness]. Then Ra said: "Put him upon his bed until he has recovered." It was Set---he has assumed form against him as a black pig; thereupon he shot a blow into his eye. Then Ra said: "The pig is an abomination to Heru." "Would that he might recover," said the gods. That is how the pig became an abomination to the gods, as well as men, for Herus' sake..."

http://www.fordham.edu/halsall/ancient/1900horuspig.asp
Also in the **Pert em Hru - Chapter 30B**
[See page 15 of the transliteration and translation]:
*http://books.google.com/books?id=SGBDAQAAIAAJ&printsec=
frontcov...*

So much for not eating the pig; I always thought that tradition belonged to the Muslims, who knew that the ancient Blacks of Kamit, or so-called Egypt, actually had a tradition of the non-consumption of the pig...and perhaps the Muslims, Jews and others got the tradition from Sweet Black Mama Africa.

In the same text Pert em Hru – chapter 30B, a portion reads:

"This chapter should be read by a person purified and cleansed, who has not eaten animal flesh or fish..."

[See page 15 of the transliteration and translation]:
*http://books.google.com/books?id=SGBDAQAAIAAJ&printsec=
frontcov...*

Nyansapo

Here, ritual purification and cleansing ('Twra' as spelled in the metutu - Dwra or Dwira as spelled in Akan) is associated with the refraining from the consumption of animal flesh and fish. (Owirafo 2014) www.odwirafo.com/Akanfo_Nanasom.html

Anthony Browder, noted Egyptologist, author and scholar, shared with me, that the priesthood of ancient Kamit did not partake of eating animals while working at the temples for several weeks at a time. He did not know if the tradition continued when the priest/priestess returned to their home.

Purification and cleansing is a ritual that many in the African centered community (Ausar Auset, Akan, Yoruba, Hebrew Israelites, etc.) still practice. For more information on how to fast, abstain and cleanse during certain cycles, see 'Fasting Options' on page 102.

A few more thoughts and facts about eating a plant-based diet:

❖ Many proclaim dead chickens are full of toxins.

❖ Animals for consumption may be routinely drugged with chemicals like arsenic and artificial hormones.

❖ Meat consumption could be considered a violence-based food source. Killing is a violent act, even if done with mercy.

❖ Animal beings suffer pain and experience fear and loss as they are being slaughtered.

❖ The animal beings experience a range of feeling and emotions as they witness and listen to other animal beings, being slaughtered.

- ❖ The American Heart Association and American Cancer Society sites state that meat, chicken, pork, eggs, and cheese cause most of our diseases.

- ❖ The eating of flesh is linked to heart disease, some cancers, and osteoporosis.

- ❖ Chicken can contain 3 times the fat as it did thirty-five years ago.

- ❖ Arsenic is a toxin to humans however it is often used in feed to promote faster growth and consequently faster profits.

- ❖ Chicken can contain a high bacterial contamination ratio.

- ❖ Calcium can be leached out of the body due to the high protein content of animal products, including milk.

- ❖ Harvard Medical School wrote that milk does not protect us from osteoporosis.

- ❖ Pesticides and herbicides are more concentrated in meat/animal dairy products because the animals eat contaminated foods and the substances become concentrated in the milk as well as the flesh.

The Journal of American Medical Association, June 3, 1961, p. 806

❖ Animal products are often loaded with antibiotics, artificial hormones, and heavy metals. These toxins are not found in plants. The question looms as to whether hormones are the causes of early pubescent development in girls and possibly the feminization of males. (Chemicals found in soft plastics and overconsumption of processed soy are also thought to imbalance hormones in males).

❖ Long term weight loss is best supported when the individual follows a plant-based diet that primarily consists of fresh foods.

❖ Meat eaters may have three times the obesity of vegetarians.

❖ Dr. Colin Campbell of Cornell University, an epidemiologist wrote, "Quite simply, the more you substitute plant foods for animal foods, the healthier you are likely to become. I now consider veganism to be the ideal diet, one that is low in fat and will substantially lower the risk of disease with no disadvantages. Vegans appear to enjoy equal or better health in comparison to vegetarians and non-vegetarians." China Study, 2005

❖ The Vegetarian Resources Group estimates that there are now more than 47 million vegetarians on the planet. Vegetarian Resource Group, http://www.vrg.org.

❖ You can be healthy without killing animals; therefore he who eats meat is doing it for the sake of one's own appetite. If you are interested in health and have a compassion for animals, then a plant-based diet is the way to go.

❖ A plant-based diet is more considerate of the limited resources of our planet. The eating of animals utilizes great amounts of energy while the animal is being raised and prepared for slaughter. The fecal matter which runs into the streams and rivers pollutes our waterways. Then the dead animal flesh must be taken to market utilizing yet another form of energy.

❖ Vegetarian comes from the Latin word *vegetus* meaning "full of life."

❖ Vedic scriptures from India stress nonviolence as the ethical foundation of vegetarianism. *Manu-samhita (Indian Law)* reads,

○ "Meat can never be obtained without injury to living creatures. Injury to sentient beings is detrimental to the attainment of heavenly bliss. Let him therefore shun the use of meat...Having well considered the disgusting origin of flesh and cruelty of fettering and slaying or corporeal being, let him entirely abstain from eating flesh."

❖ These ancient teachings were introduced to the world through the Hare Krishna movement founded by Srila Prabhupada and to many in the Black community by Swami Krisnapada.

❖ Traditional Buddhism advocated the doctrine of Ahimasa or nonviolence to all beings.

Nyansapo

❖ St. Jerome who wrote the Latin version of the Bible wrote,
  ○ "...a plant-based diet was the best for a life devoted to the pursuit of wisdom."

❖ St. Benedict, who founded the Benedictine Order in A.D. 529, stipulated vegan foods for the monks.

❖ In the sixth century B.C. Pythagoras is given credit for the hygienic nature of a plant-based diet.

❖ St. Francis of Assisi was an early follower of the vegetarian way of life, as were Leonardo Da Vinci and Isaac Newton.

❖ Isaiah 66: 3
  ○ He that killeth an ox (cow) is as if he slew a man.

❖ Genesis 1: 11-13
  ○ And God said, "Let the earth bring forth grass, the herb (vegetable) yielding seed, and the fruit tree yielding fruit after his own kind, whose seed is in itself, upon the earth" and it was so...and God saw that it was good. And the evening and the morning were the third day.

❖ Daniel 1: 8
  ○ "But Daniel purposed in his heart that he would not defile himself with the portion of the King's meat....

Akofena

Courage

Slam Dunk Veggie

After reading and studying and listening to talks on vegetarianism, the underlying consensus may be just stop eating the stuff! By the "stuff" I am referring to the five whites, the processed junk food, the dead animal products, the fried foods, GMOs, and the other detrimental foods outlined in this book. Clean out your kitchen and refrigerator and replace the items you discard with life giving foods. Some people are able do this; I could not. I call it slam dunk veg! Bam, I am a vegetarian! Just do it today. If you backslide, don't beat yourself up. Get back on the greens as soon as possible and begin your journey again. Have a support system of other plant eaters in place when you fall off the green juice.

The internet makes this easy. One source is Elaine Rice-Fells' rawsoul@yahoogroups.com, and rawsoul-rainbow colors on facebook.com. Another source you can consider joining is black vegetarian societies which are easy to search for by city. But a physical support system is great to have because we are humans and connecting is basic to our existence. I encourage you to find local health food stores or vegetarian websites that are African owned. Surround yourself with people who will not judge you, who will love you, who will support, and encourage you on your journey. Expect the biological family to tease you...no worries! In the end, they will be running to you for information and suggestions in the face of sickness, disease, and scary diagnoses.

Many people call themselves vegetarian, but they are still ingesting flesh, which is a contradiction. It is normal to take steps in this transformation process, but to call yourself a vegetarian is a stretch. Perhaps one could refer to oneself as an **evolving** or **transitioning** vegetarian. I would recommend one to eat primarily a plant-based diet and work toward being a vegetarian/vegan or raw foodist.

What Kind of Vegetarian are You?

Fruitarian	Eats only uncooked fruits, nuts, and seeds
Live/Raw vegan	Eat vegan foods that are uncooked
Vegans	Do not eat any animals or animal by-products
Vegetarians	Do not eat animals
Lacto Vegetarians	Do not eat animal flesh, but eat dairy products
Lacto-Ovo Vegetarians	Do not eat animal flesh, but they eat dairy and eggs
Ovo-vegetarians	Do not eat animal flesh but they eat eggs

Thee are many other categories including pescatarian and polo vegetarian. For the purpose of this work, we are trying to free your mind, then your behind from flesh and flesh by-products step by step; therefore, we are only going to discuss the top four vegetarians on the above chart.

Any progress that one makes on this path is beneficial and will impact one's health and/or energy level. The most important point is to always keep taking the steps. Always keep taking the steps, you may never arrive at the destination. Embrace the process! Building a strong repertoire of knowledge is one of the most critical life changes you can make, impacting your health and the health of your posse.

Let me share with you some ways to make the transition and you determine your own personal dietary journey to better health!

Eliminate the Five Whites

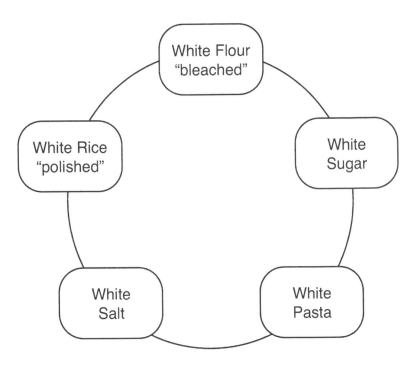

The Step Pyramid Method

Start at the bottom and work your way up. Give yourself a timeline to be at your next step of toxic food elimination. Listen to your body, mind, and spirit. It will help you in this process of letting go of foods that no longer serve you. Before you start on this transition plan you might want to consider eliminating cigarettes, alcohol, drugs, fast foods, refined salt, bleached processed flours and grains, soda, and other sugary drinks. All of these products will compromise your health, as they continue to make the corporations who are selling addiction and illness, materially rich.

Increase water intake, buy 100% fruit juice and dilute it with water by 50% prior to drinking. Once you get used to this, increase the percentage of water to juice and reduce the glycemic load of sugar...cancer loves sugar!

If it says 100% natural, that doesn't mean it is all fruit. There is lots of food industry trickery at play. Read the ingredients before you put it in the cart. No sugar, fructose, dextrose—you want just the fruit. I look for 100% & organic on the label. Later, you can get your own juicer, start juicing at home, and begin an even deeper healing.

So → Let's → Step →

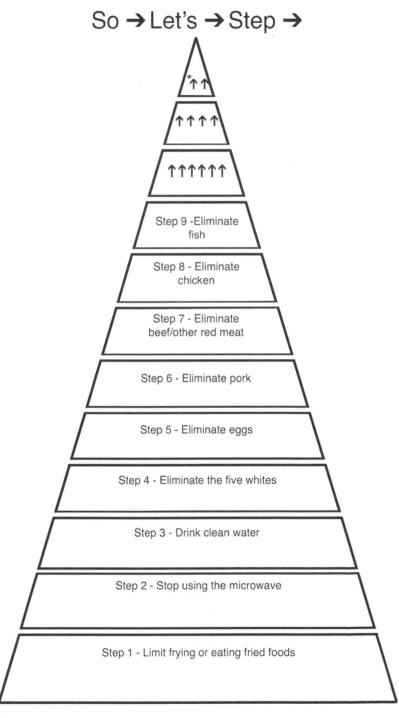

↑↑

↑↑↑↑

↑↑↑↑↑↑

Step 9 - Eliminate fish

Step 8 - Eliminate chicken

Step 7 - Eliminate beef/other red meat

Step 6 - Eliminate pork

Step 5 - Eliminate eggs

Step 4 - Eliminate the five whites

Step 3 - Drink clean water

Step 2 - Stop using the microwave

Step 1 - Limit frying or eating fried foods

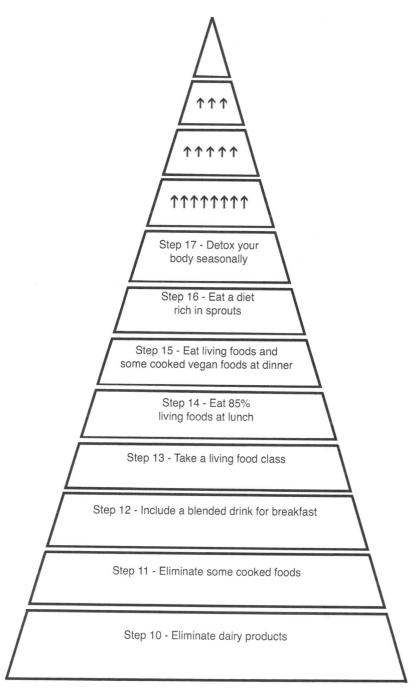

↑ ↑ ↑

↑ ↑ ↑ ↑ ↑

↑ ↑ ↑ ↑ ↑ ↑ ↑ ↑

Step 17 - Detox your body seasonally

Step 16 - Eat a diet rich in sprouts

Step 15 - Eat living foods and some cooked vegan foods at dinner

Step 14 - Eat 85% living foods at lunch

Step 13 - Take a living food class

Step 12 - Include a blended drink for breakfast

Step 11 - Eliminate some cooked foods

Step 10 - Eliminate dairy products

Step 1   Limit frying or eating fried foods

Step 2   Consider not using the microwave oven.
                It changes the cellular structure of food

Step 3   Drink clean water—not tap water without
                filtration. Consider a Reverse Osmosis home
                filtration unit.

Step 4   Eliminate the whites: white sugar, white pota-
                toes, white (processed) salt, white flour, white
                rice, white pasta and most processed foods
                (foods in cans, boxes – foods that are not alive).

Step 5   Eliminate eggs from your diet and products
                made with eggs. Think of it as chicken ovum
                without sperm. Do you really need a chicken
                ovum???

Step 6   Eliminate the lowly pig from your plate.

Step 7   Eliminate beef and other red blooded animals.
                Okay, okay I know you might be having trouble
                at this stage. So, visit a flesh processing factory,
                commonly called a meat packaging facility and
                just observe (remember my visit at the age of
                16). Then visit the rivers where these compa-
                nies dump the resulting waste. Make sure you
                hold your nose. You will have a transforming
                image etched in the recesses of your mind for-
                ever. Conversely, just do a week of YouTube Uni-
                versity and put slaughter houses in the search
                engine. That might be enough to jolt your spirit
                back to nature. Also one could stand outside the

butcher's corner in your local store. If the stench doesn't get to you first, the eerie feeling of coldness and death looming like an evil cloud will. But to hear the animal scream and cry when they are actually murdered is the real haunting and revolting part and may shake you out of the sanitized world view that we have been fed about eating slaughtered animals.

Step 8   Eliminate chicken from your plate. These animals may carry a high degree of bacteria and are injected with drugs while in human captivity awaiting their death sentence, so that they can make an appearance on your plate. Have mercy on the creatures of this planet. They deserve a life. Perhaps if we can stop killing the animals, we can move to stop the killing of humans and move humanity to a higher plane. Peace on Earth 365, a planet without war.

Step 9   Eliminate fish. While you are working on this step, first stop eating bottom fish that eat the garbage of the rivers and oceans, commonly referred to as scavengers (ex:catfish). Stop eating the shellfish. Until you can work it out at this level, eat the small fish that primarily eat vegetation. Consider sardines, I know they are not sexy, but during this transition time, come out of your comfort zone. On special occasions you might want to go for salmon, granted not a small fish, however a very virtuous one in terms of nutritional qualities. Wild is the best. Many years ago the Black Muslims sold a whiting fish from unpolluted waters. If you still feel the need to eat fish, eat only from unpolluted sources if you can find any. (Salmon sold in USA is soon to be GMO. It appears Monsanto has the Statue of Liberty by it's ovaries).

Step 10   Eliminate dairy products from your diet. Learn to make your non-dairy milk and cheese, or buy vegan products. At this point, you can refer to yourself as a vegan. But don't stop, keep going— never stop growing/glowing and going forward in your life. If you back slide, no biggie, just don't do it all the time.

Step 11   Eliminate some of the cooked food in your diet and start eating more living or raw/fresh foods. Raw or living foods are fresh fruits and vegetables that have not been cooked by anything but the sun. Learn to juice and learn to make blended drinks. Try to eat at least 50% living food at every meal working toward a "high live" diet where you will be eating 70 to 80% live foods daily. A high live diet will keep the glow in your aura and your skin. You will appear youthful, which makes so much sense, as now you are consuming life and foods full of life, so your appearance becomes vibrant and healthy.

Step 12   Consider making a blended fruit drink for breakfast. Add some organic greens and non-soy protein powder. Another option can be a nut milk smoothie as part of breakfast. (NOTE: Blended drinks are foods that are blended in a blender, not juiced, and then consumed. They provide all the fiber from the plant. This encourages a kind of roto-rooter action in the bowels. When you get to this stage invest in a plunger, you are going to need it.)

Step 13   Take a living foods class, workshop, or a Detox group fast. Keep learning! Books are also an option. Start making what you have learned.

Step 14   85% living foods at lunch.

Step 15   Eat living food and some cooked vegan foods at dinner.

Step 16   Include a diet that is rich in sprouts. Use them in your blended drinks and on salads and wraps. Sprouts are packed with enzymes and easily digested. They pack a lot of power for very little effort on our bodies' behalf.

Step 17   Learn to detox your body at home and with a professional on a seasonal basis. This might include liquid diets, enemas, colon hydrotherapy, steam sauna, infrared sauna, ozone, aqua chi, clay, brushing, inversion therapy, juice feast etc.

Visit the HealingTree Detox Day Spa for an in-depth consultation or detox spa session.

The following chart will give you a base plan to transition from a vegetarian primarily cooked palate to a raw or living food palate. Make these charts work for you, they are not set in stone. Planning is crucial in navigating a plant based diet. You will back slide when you have not planned and prepared what you are going to eat the next day or the next week. Drink a glass of water when you are being tempted to eat something that is not for your highest good. This will give you time to rethink your actions. While at the same time, giving you a feeling of fullness.

Healthy eating is truly an art. It requires a little getting used to in the beginning but it is so worth it to live a healthy life, free from disease, excessive drugs, unnecessary medical interventions and low energy.

Although a plant based diet is not a magic bullet and a cure all, it will help you to stay in good health along exercise, fasting, detoxing , sunlight and sleep on a regular basis. Nubians don't run from the Sun, we run to it! The Sun loves us, we are naturally responsive to it; it is the life- giver to almost everything on this planet! I try to keep my melanin pumped from spring to fall. This aids in having a natural glow of health and vitality.

Akofena

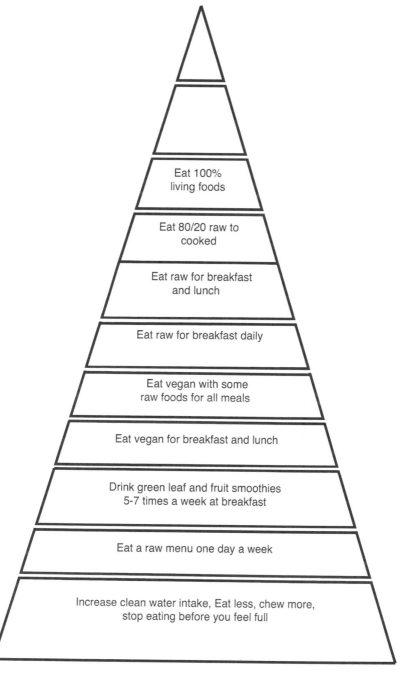

Eat 100%
living foods

Eat 80/20 raw to
cooked

Eat raw for breakfast
and lunch

Eat raw for breakfast daily

Eat vegan with some
raw foods for all meals

Eat vegan for breakfast and lunch

Drink green leaf and fruit smoothies
5-7 times a week at breakfast

Eat a raw menu one day a week

Increase clean water intake, Eat less, chew more,
stop eating before you feel full

Other Transitional Methods to Consider

➤ Consider eating a plant based diet for one day a week increasing the number of days as your body becomes accustomed to the foods and as your knowledge of plant-based recipes increases.

➤ Consider eating raw all meals with one serving of cooked veggies or soaked and sprouted grains.

➤ (I have found it is much easier to eat raw/live during the warm seasons if you live in the cold regions. Take the weather into account and shift as the seasons change. Eat more fruits from spring to fall. Try this if you need to drop 10-20 pounds. All foods with seeds are considered fruit. (Do not eat seedless fruits. They may impact your fertility).

The next chart will help with step by step suggestions to a raw or living food diet which is a diet that is primarily uncooked or cooked at low temperatures or in a dehydrator. It can also be used as a detox guide. For example, if for some time you have been eating a 50/50 diet, then to detox move to one of the steps above that. When finished you can return to 50/50 or stay at the higher step.

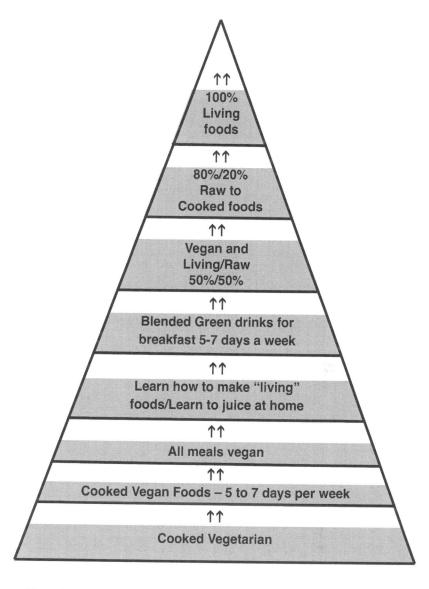

(Read the chart from the bottom and work your way up!!)

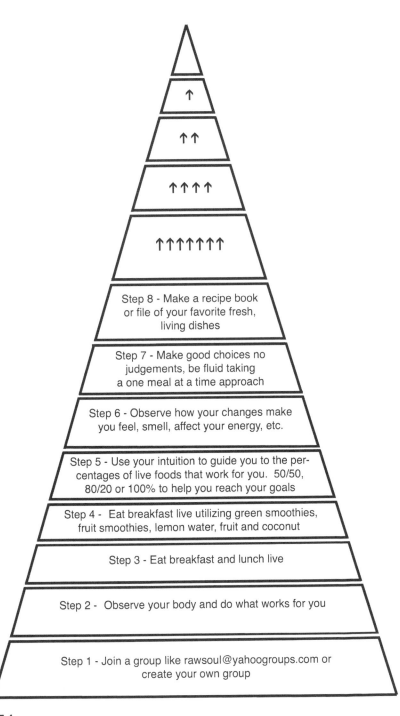

↑

↑ ↑

↑ ↑ ↑ ↑

↑ ↑ ↑ ↑ ↑ ↑ ↑

Step 8 - Make a recipe book
or file of your favorite fresh,
living dishes

Step 7 - Make good choices no
judgements, be fluid taking
a one meal at a time approach

Step 6 - Observe how your changes make
you feel, smell, affect your energy, etc.

Step 5 - Use your intuition to guide you to the per-
centages of live foods that work for you. 50/50,
80/20 or 100% to help you reach your goals

Step 4 - Eat breakfast live utilizing green smoothies,
fruit smoothies, lemon water, fruit and coconut

Step 3 - Eat breakfast and lunch live

Step 2 - Observe your body and do what works for you

Step 1 - Join a group like rawsoul@yahoogroups.com or
create your own group

Akofena

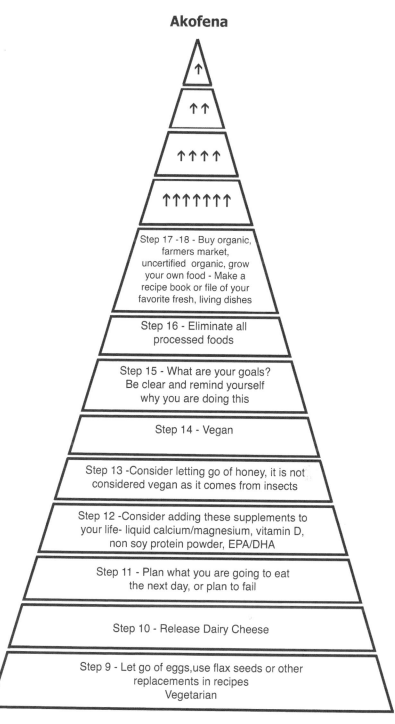

↑

↑ ↑

↑ ↑ ↑ ↑

↑↑↑↑↑↑↑

Step 17 -18 - Buy organic,
farmers market,
uncertified organic, grow
your own food - Make a
recipe book or file of your
favorite fresh, living dishes

Step 16 - Eliminate all
processed foods

Step 15 - What are your goals?
Be clear and remind yourself
why you are doing this

Step 14 - Vegan

Step 13 -Consider letting go of honey, it is not
considered vegan as it comes from insects

Step 12 -Consider adding these supplements to
your life- liquid calcium/magnesium, vitamin D,
non soy protein powder, EPA/DHA

Step 11 - Plan what you are going to eat
the next day, or plan to fail

Step 10 - Release Dairy Cheese

Step 9 - Let go of eggs,use flax seeds or other
replacements in recipes
Vegetarian

Consider meditating and praying about how you should go about making the change. For example:

Thank you God, bless me with the strength and will-power to make enlightened changes and choices in my diet. For this I do give thanks. Amen, Amen, Amen!

Ankoben

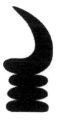

Vigilance and Wariness

Backing up from Chemicals and Devitalized Foods The Battle Cry for Your Health

Organic vs. Conventional Fruits and Vegetables

As a transitioning vegetarian/vegan, try to purchase your foods organic when possible. Conventional fruits and vegetables often contain herbicides and pesticides that impact your health. This list shows you the items that you must purchase organic and the items that you do not have to purchase organic. The list is not conclusive, but will point you in the right direction.

Fruits and Veggies that do not have to be purchased organic:

Avocados
Pineapple*
Cabbage
Sweet peas (frozen)
Onions
Asparagus
Mango* could be GMO
Papaya* could be GMO
Kiwi
Eggplant
Grapefruit
Cantaloupe (domestic)
Cauliflower
Sweet potatoes
Broccoli
Watermelon

*The starred foods may be genetically modified depending on the country or origin.

Fruits and Veggies that should always be purchased organic:

Apples
Strawberries
Blueberries
Blackberries
Cranberries
Grapes
Leafy Greens
Corn

Some people wonder if purchasing the more expensive organic food items is really meaningful. Take a look at the pesticide chart below. These conventional foods were found to have a variety of pesticides in them. (This list may have some omissions).

This list will get you started. Remember to use suspect foods in moderation or avoid all together. When you purchase organic foods, you avoid pesticides, herbicides, and GMO crops.

The this chart gives you a breakdown of how many pesticides are found in conventional foods. It does not include paraffin other toxics variables.

• FOOD ITEM	NO. OF PESTICIDES FOUND IN NON-ORGANIC FOOD ITEM
MISCELLANEOUS	
•	
• Milk	10
• Coffee	12
•	
VEGETABLES	
• Celery	64
• Kale	42
• Pepper	49
• Potatoes	37
• Spinach	48
• Carrots	26
• Green Leafy	51
•	
FRUITS	
• Blackberries	52
• Cherries	42
• Grapes	34
• Nectarines	33
• Peaches	42
• Strawberries	59

www.ewg.org

GMOs

If you are a snacker, and most of us are, you are going to want to buy organic corn or potato chips. Why? Another nasty three letter word, GMO. Ok, it's not really a word; it's an acronym that stands for **Genetically Modified Organism** and is used to refer to plants and animals whose genetic material has been artificially manipulated. That means companies like Monsanto have tried to change Mother Nature in the laboratory. GMO seeds including corn end up in many foods, such as tortillas chips, corn chips, corn syrup, corn meal, and even **animal feed**-- giving you yet another reason not to eat them animals

So all packaged foods could be potentially laden with GMOs, as they generally contain a version of corn, corn oil, corn flour, corn meal or potato starch. Be very wary of foods that have soy as it is one of the major products known as a GMO. Additionally soy is known to disrupt the hormones and can impact the thyroid adversely. However we are told that tempeh is safe, hopefully that remains true; if not, we may need to figure out how to make our own. When you buy papaya make sure it is not from Hawaii. They too produce GMOs along with zucchini and sweet corn. The American government does not require labeling of GMO produce, so you must, must buy these corn products. And prayerfully they have not lied and it really is organic. Of course you could grow your own! GMO foods are thought to cause infertility, leaky gut, and allergies to name a few. GMOs are banned in 26 countries including Ghana.

Sweeteners/MSG/Oils

Canola Oil – Con-nola is a better name for this industrial oil. Yes, it does have some beneficial qualities but they do not out-weigh its toxic hemagglutinins, and glycocides. The naysayers suggests that it causes mad cow disease, nervous system imbalances and disorders, clumping of blood cells and depression. It's off my list. It is made from the hybridization of the **rapeseed**, which is considered toxic due to uric acid. Do your research, but for me and mine, it's a no.

High Fructose Corn Syrup – Follow this ingredient all the way to diabetes, liver conditions, aka fatty liver issues and much, much more. It is found in most soda pop, teas, juices, candy, cookies and the stuff you feed your kids 'cause you just didn't know any better.

Dextrose – It's a sugar/glucose, often in chemical form. Our bodies are meant for food, not all these chemicals masquerading as food! Too much **sug**ar will make your blood move slow and thick. Then you'll be overweight and maybe get diabetes, or just ADHD, or rotten teeth or muscle weakness or mood swings, or a sugar addiction. Need more info? Read *Sugar Blues*. by William Duffy. **Sug** (sugar) is a sweet/rotten devil. It will prostitute your health by making your system an available candidate for diseases like cancer. Want a more scientific perspective? Google the side effects of sugar, artificial sweeteners. In the meantime, stay away from all ingredients that end in -ose!!

Brown sugar – nothing more than colored white sugar with the same blues. Not to be confused with raw natural sugar, perhaps made from dates. Use organic cane brown sugar as a substitute.

Artificial sweeteners – There are a host of scientific reasons not to ingest artificial sweeteners, including brain tumors, seizures, heart attacks, kidney and liver dysfunction,blurred vision,weight gain, and allergic reactions.GMO corn products are often used in the production of some of these products, as well as mercury and chlorine, read Sweet Deception by Dr. Mercola for more information.

MSG – monosodium glutamate, this flavoring was created in Japan by Kikunae Ikeda. This laboratory food enhancer is found in the seasoning Accent, canned foods, crackers, soy sauce, and numerous other foods. This ingredient is known to over-excite your brain cells. The FDA states the following about MSG:

> *"Studies have shown that the body uses glutamate, an amino acid, as a nerve impulse transmitter in the brain and that there are glutamate-responsive tissues in other parts of the body, as well.*
>
> *Abnormal function of glutamate receptors has been linked with certain neurological diseases, such as Alzheimer's disease and Huntington's chorea. Injections of glutamate in laboratory animals have resulted in damage to nerve cells in the brain."*

U.S. Food and Drug Administration "FDA and Monosodium Glutamate (MSG)" August 31, 1995

Some suggest that the use of MSG could result in
- Cardiac Arrhythmia
- Obesity

- Fatigue
- Disorientation
- Depression
- Eye problems

Short term reactions, to name only a few, may include the following:

- Numbness
- Tingling
- Chest pain
- Rapid heartbeat
- General weakness

Want more info? Read Dr Blaylock's book, *Excitotoxin, The Taste that Kills.* You don't need a degree to know it's a bad mama jama to be avoided!!!

It is now imported into West Africa, and is purchased in the local markets by the pound to Africans. I saw this in Tema Market.

MSG is often found in the following:

- Hydrolyzed Protein
- Hydrolyzed Vegetable Protein
- Plant protein Extract
- Sodium Caseinate
- Calcium Caseinate

- Yeast Extract
- Textured Protein
- Autolyzed Yeast

- ❖ Hydrolyzed Oat Flour
- ❖ Corn oil
- ❖ Malt Extract Malt flavoring
- ❖ Bouillon
- ❖ Broth
- ❖ Stock
- ❖ Flavoring
- ❖ Natural Flavors/flavoring
- ❖ Seasoning
- ❖ Spices

Food additives that MAY contain MSG or excitotoxins:
- ❖ Carrageen
- ❖ Enzymes
- ❖ Soy Protein Concentrate
- ❖ Soy Protein Isolate
- ❖ Whey Protein Concentrated
- ❖ Protease Enzymes
- ❖ Aspartame is an extreme source of excitotoxins
- ❖ Found in NutraSweet & Equal, Diet soft drinks, sugar free gums, Crystal Light, children's medications

Oils are one of the primary foods where GMOs have found a home. Fast food restaurants use them all day. Ask them what kind of oil their food is cooked in. They will tell you a vegetable oil. Then ask them to show you the container so you can read it for yourself. All vegetable oils are not wholesome—due to processing and GMO's. Nuf said?

Hydrogenated oils are almost as bad as the death penalty. Due to the negative impact they have on the liver and the digestive system.

Oils not to use - remember they are cheap cause they will make you ill in time, don't be tempted homey/sistah mama!

> **Corn oil**
> **Soy oil**
> **Canola oil**
> **ANY hydrogenated oil**
> **Trans fats**

People and corporations are banking on you making stupid un-informed choices about your health in your buying habits. They are making millions from selling you bad/unhealthy food. Then when you get sick they sell you drugs, medical appointments and procedures, never telling you that what you eat is slowly killing your black or brown or beige behind. So get down with this so you can help yourself, your family, and others. Together we will win, *Pumoja tu tashinda!*

The queen of oils is most definitely coconut oil. This oil is great for the skin, heart, brain, immune system and the thyroid. If you want to jump start your metabolism, coconut oil is the way to go. Taking a tablespoon a day is said to boost the metabolism. Who knew that eating a fat could help to lose fat. If you ate animal fat in this method you would have heart complications in a hurry!

Coconut oil is also said to help destroy viruses as well as have antibiotic characteristics. Don't believe me, do your own research, you'll see. While doing your research, check the westonaprice.org. They have an excellent article on oils entitled "the skinny on fats!"

For many years we were told in the West to avoid the oils out of the tropics, specifically coconut and palm. We were told that the saturated oils were not healthy for our hearts. Instead,we were directed to refined oils and seed oils. Now we are being told that coconut and palm oils are ok! Yes I know it is confusing, that is why it is extremely helpful to have someone in your family or circle, who is up on the latest food and natural medicine research as it is ever-changing. So just to keep it simple.

Best Oils to Use
  - ➤ Unprocessed Coconut oils – preferably organic and cold pressed
  - ➤ Unprocessed Red Palm oils – organic and cold pressed
  - ➤ Extra Virgin olive oils – in dark bottles
  - ➤ Flax Seed oil for uncooked foods

If you are cooking at high temperatures, tropical oils are better to use, extra virgin olive oil is best for living foods and low heat.

Read your food labels and avoid packaged foods with oils that are not good for you. Case in point, I was ready to buy some vegan cheese, I flipped over the package to read the ingredients and the first item listed was canola oil (con-ola). I threw it down and walked away. (If you know better, do better.) In the long run, all these changes will bring you better health and longevity. A plant based diet is not a guarantee against dis-ease (I use this word interchangeably with disease to reflect that the body is in an uneasy state) or a cure all, but paired with movement it is a healthy lifestyle.

ACID/ALKALINE BALANCE

From http://www.crossroads-chiropractic.com/?p=411

If you are eating/drinking a green drink daily and eating mostly vegetables, you won't have to worry about keeping your body alkaline. Foods fall in one category or the other. Our bodies are mostly Alkaline. When we keep our bodies in the alkaline range it is very difficult for disease to overtake us. Yet when we become too acidic, the disease can flourish within us. **Meats** are acidic, some vegetables are categorized as acidic like some grains and beans. I always try to eat lots of green veggies and green leaves. This will help you to stay on the alkaline side.

Ankoben

Queen Afua taught that many men are giving their Queens womb problems because they have acidic semen. Sugar, alcohol, drugs, pharmaceuticals, certain waters, and cigarettes create an acidic internal environment. But their Queens may be making the situation worse with the five whites or hanging onto the chicken. So eat your greens. If you are on the road, then take green supplements like spirulina, chlorella or African moringa. There are volumes written on the subject, this is just meant to be an overview, just enough to tease your curiosity to go and read more on this subject.

Below is a simple chart of foods and their acid and alkaline levels—the lower number refers to a more acidic level. The following acid levels are an approximation. Some foods are on one level when first eaten, then on another after digestion. But this will give you a general idea and you will understand on a deeper level why we stay away from the **five whites**.

- Colas 1.0
- Soft drinks artificially sweetened 1.0
- Sugar 1.0
- Liquor 1.0-2.0
- Coffee 1.5
- Salt Refined 1.5
- Wheat Refined 1.5
- White Rice 1.5
- Cereal Corn 2.5
- Meat 2.5
- Fried Potato Chips 3.0
- Chicken & Fish 3.0

- Prescribed drugs are normally highly acidic
- Melons 7.0
- Asparagus 6.5
- Pineapple 6.5
- Fresh Fruit Juices 6.5
- Avocados 6.0
- Citrus Fruits 6.0
- Most Vegetables 5.0-6.0
- Potatoes with Skin 5.5
- Almonds 5.0

Some experts indicate that we should be striving for 80/20 ratio of alkaline to acid ratio with our daily diet. Persons who are too acidic may find themselves with headaches, pains, and problems with sleep – because of too much build-up of acid in the system. Acidic salts, which can build up in the body over decades can lead to bone problems like osteoporosis.

- Eating and drinking at the same time will increase your acid load.
- Measure your saliva or urine with ph stick and adjust your lifestyle.
- Good food combining helps to reduce your acid load.
- Infections have a hard time existing in an alkaline environment.

(See why back in the day we could only have sweets on Sundays!! And why we ate only a little bit of meat!! This was a blessing in the disguise of poverty).

Some of our activities can be categorized as acid like or alkaline like. It is believed that the alkaline individual is more peaceful than an acid person.

Alkaline-producing activities/emotions: Meditation, Prayer, Peace, Happiness, Kindness, Love Neutral pH 7.0 - Healthy Body Saliva pH Range is between 6.4 to 6.8 (on your pH test strip)

Acid producing activities/emotions: Overwork, Anger, Fear, Jealousy & Stress.

This information will help you to monitor your eating habits. We often eat not because we are hungry, but due to emotional issues, like stress, disappointment, anger, including indirect anger. Learn to listen to your body and its call for food. Often the call is for clean water, so go there first. Wait, and if you still feel hungry, after 30 minutes, eat. Remember information is power; refer to this chart as needed.

EXAMPLES OF ACID AND ALKALINE FOODS

ACID FORMING FOODS	ALKALINE FORMING FOODS
(Diet should be 20% Acid Forming Foods)	*(Diet should be 80% Alkaline Forming Foods)*
Junk Food	
Meat/Animal Products/Eggs	
Nuts & Legumes	*Green leafy, the darker the better*
Alcohol and Nicotine	
Synthetic Foods	
Grains	*Most Fruits and Vegetables*
Dairy Products	
Processed Salt*	

*Salt is acid, some salts (Himalayan Sea Salt - HSS) are better than others.

Habitual eating of certain types of foods may have an emotional component. I've included the E.A.F. chart so you can see what perhaps the underlying causes of food cravings/addictions are. You might need support or even counseling around certain food choices. Emotional eating can be addressed through a variety of modalities including supplements, auricular acupuncture, breath work, and Emotional Freedom Technique (EFT), to name a few techniques.

Snack Food Addictions

Type	Emotional Addictive Factor
1. Bready	■ Relieves feelings of insecurity and soothes dissatisfaction
2. Chewy	■ Relieves tension/stress and need to slowdown and unwind
3. Creamy	■ Helps satisfy need to be nurtured and comforted
4. Crunchy	■ Helps release anxiety, pressure
5. Salty	■ Redirects anger, frustration, violence
6. Sugary	■ Helps satisfy need to give and/or receive love

Okodee Mmowere

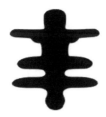

Strength, Bravery, Power

Common Elements
Missing in American Diets

Many of us are deficient in vitamins and minerals. If you are knowledgeable of what your body is lacking, then it is best to use a food source to alleviate the problem. In dire situations this is not advised, and one must supplement with high quality vitamins immediately. Remember to chew well and chew until the food is liquid, your stomach does not have teeth. Eating fast and talking while eating, also not wise. The following chart will provide you with a list of foods to eat when one has a deficiency or to prevent a deficiency.

Where to Find Your Minerals

Mineral	Purpose	Food Sources
Calcium	Bones, Skeletal structure, teeth,	Dandelion greens Nuts & Seeds Carrot Juice Broccoli Wheat grass
Silicone	Hair, elasticity of skin	Dandelion Yucca Leaves Asparagus Cauliflower Nuts & Seeds
Iodine	Feeds thyroid, controls weight and metabolism	Sea veggies Black walnut Garlic Onions
Sodium	Fluid Balance Muscle contraction Nerve Transmission	Sunflower Parsley Licorice Celery Cucumber Strawberries Okra Dandelion Sesame Seeds Red Cabbage Figs Watercress

Okodee Mmowere

Where to find your minerals continued...

Mineral	Purpose	Food Sources
Potassium	Fluid Balance Muscle Contraction Nerve Transmission	Kelp Parsley Ginger Red Pepper Banana Raisins Potato Peel Bitter Greens Grains
Iron	Energy metabolism Carries oxygen	Kelp Black cherries Dried Fruits Strawberries Black Strap Molasses
B-12	Helps with cell division and red blood cells	MISO Sea Veggies Alfalfa Ginseng Nutritional yeast (organic)

HEALTH DEPLETING AGENTS

The following list of substances will destroy or compromise your health if abused. They should not be used if one is feeling weak or if one is working toward vibrancy in health, these items should be used in moderation or not at all.

- ❖ Coffee/caffeine depletes → iron, potassium, calcium, iodine
- ❖ Alcohol depletes → potassium
- ❖ Red meats deplete → potassium
- ❖ Excessive use of synthetic laxatives depletes 'vitamin A, vitamin D, & vitamin E→
- ❖ Salt and/or sugar depletes → silicon
- ❖ Food additives deplete → iron
- ❖ Food preservatives deplete →
- ❖ ANTACIDS deplete → sodium
- ❖ Junk foods deplete → B12

Radiation from television, X-rays, power lines deplete → iodine

Discover what you can eat that is good for you! If you are a newbie, take this list to the store with you when you go shopping. The list is especially helpful when you want to make your favorite dish in a healthy way. Granted, it may not taste the same but at least, it will not make you sick, Slick! Healthy eating is an acquired taste, so hang with me Shorty.

Healthy Substitutes

Sugar

Stevia, agave, maple syrup, rice syrup, date sugar, dried fruit w/o sugar, raw honey(not vegan), ripe banana

**Animal Fats
Margarine**

Use organic cold pressed – no saturated or hydrogenated: Coconut, Extra Virgin Olive, Safflower, Grapeseed, Peanut, Red Palm

Salt (not a food)

Sea Salt, Himalayan Salt, Celery/Celery Seed, Sea Vegetables, Kelp, Nori, Dulse, Salt substitutes, miso.

Eggs

Flax seed whole or ground placed in water will thicken water(strain seeds out), chia seed water, agar-agar

Animal Protein

Soaked nuts, Organic nut butters, nut milk, non-soy vegetable protein, tempeh, sprouts, lentils, small sprouted beans, adzuki, mung, navy beans (eat beans raw or cook in slow cooker.)
Power Meal protein powder, Moringa, Spirulina, hemp powder or seeds, chia seeds, freekeh, coconuts

Healthy Substitutes... continued

Enriched White Flour — Millet flour, sprouted grains that have been ground, spelt amaranth, wheat berries, oat, gout, rye, buckwheat, sprouted bread, rice tortillas

White Rice — Brown rice, basmati rice, Millet, Quinoa, Kamut, Sprouted grains or product, freekeh, mung thread, sea kelp noodles, chia fettuccine

Thickeners — Arrowroot, kudzu, gari, agar-agar, Chia seed, Flax seed placed in water will thicken water(strain seeds out), blueberries, apples, parsley, ground nuts & ogbono seeds

Milk — Homemade nut milk, coconut milk, commercial rice milk (use sparingly), seed milks (pumpkin and sesame seed, make your own when possible)

Chocolate — Carob, Cacao

Onions and Garlic — Asafoetida (Hing)

Baking Soda — Non-Aluminum Baking Soda

Cookware — Stainless steel or glass

Toxic Internal Environment

The causes of disease can often be a mix of nutritional, mental, emotional and environmental factors. The constant buildup of everyday toxins in our tissue can lead to an unbalanced and unhealthy internal environment. Lifestyle conditions can also play a role in today's culture, for example women often use tight undergarments which may stagnate the lymph flow and add to a toxic condition. Here is a list of factors that contribute to toxic internal environments:

Pesticides & Chemicals in food

Over Cooking

Eating fast

Unbalanced diet

Constipation

Pollution in the air, water, and land

Chemicals in household products

Stagnant lymphatic system

Stress

Lack of exercise

Nutritional Deficiencies

Food storage

Poor soil

Refined foods
(see the Five Whites)

Too much Cooked foods

Weak assimilation

Weak digestion

Lack of Love

Negative state of being

Poor food combining

With a plant based diet you will be eating foods easy to digest, foods that will not clog your system with excess waste and foods that are nutrient rich in enzymes, vitamins, and mineral content. Many foods will be uncooked, which will aid the individual in assimilation and digestion.

Using the Glycemic Index to Choose Appropriate Foods

The Glycemic Index is very helpful in choosing foods, especially if one is pre-diabetic or diabetic. The glycemic index (GI) is a scale which measures how quickly carbohydrates in various foods raise glucose levels in the blood. Choose low glycemic foods to stay well and healthy. Use fruit that are low on the glycemic index when making smoothies on a daily basis. This is not the full index. You can pull up a more comprehensive version online. But it is not rocket science— starches and carbs are high on the sugar table. Foods like breads, pastas, rice, potatoes, sugars and starchy vegetables are heavier on the sugar load. So if you are diabetic or want to avoid becoming one exclude these items from your diet. Remember sweet/acid are often the item which can set the stage to illness and disease. I am going to say this twice because diabetes is running rampant in our communities. You don't **GET** diabetes you EAT **into a** diabetic condition. Read and reread this section so you can help someone and yourself.

Glycemic Index Levels and Ranges

Low GI – 55 or less
Mid-range GI – 56 – 69
High GI – 70 – 99
Glucose - 100

GRAINS & RICE	FOODS FROM GRAINS
Amaranth, popped - 97	Cereal, oats - 77
Barley - 22–50	Linguine - 43–53
Barley - 37–48	Macaroni - 45–48
Buckwheat - 45–51	Macaroni and cheese - 64
Buckwheat - 63	Porridge, oats, raw - 75
Couscous - mid	Porridge, oats, raw, rolled - 58–69
Millet, various - 71–107	Spaghetti, various - 58–68
Oat bran, raw - 57–59	Spaghetti, white - 27–53
Quinoa, boiled - 53	Spaghetti, wholemeal - 32–42
Rice, basmati - 57–69	Tortilla, corn - 78
Rice, basmati - 65	Tortillas, corn - 39–52
Rice, brown - 50	Tortillas, wheat - 28–30
Rice, brown - 66	
Rice, brown - 80	
Rye - 29–39	
Wheat - 90	
Wheat, whole - 30–48	

BREADS	FRUITS AND DRIED FRUITS
Bread, barley flour - 67	Apples, raw - 28–44
Bread, barley kernel, various kinds - 27–48	Banana, raw - 70
	Bananas, over-ripe - 48–52

BREADS	FRUITS AND DRIED FRUITS
Bread, barley, whole meal - 43–53	Bananas, raw - 46
Bread, barley, whole meal - 57–67	Grapes, raw - 23–49
Bread, cracked wheat kernel - 58	Kiwi fruits - 58
Bread, fruit and cinnamon - 71	Mangoes - 60
Bread, honey and oats - 55	Mangoes, raw - 41–51
Bread, multi-grain - 43	Oranges, raw - 31–51
Bread, multi-grain, gluten-free - 79	Papayas - 60
Bread, oat bran - 44–50	Pineapples, raw - 66
Bread, oats - 65	Plums, raw - 24–53
Bread, pita - 56–69	Prunes, pitted - 29
Bread, rice - 61	Strawberries, raw - 40
Bread, rye - 63	Sultanas - 56–58
Bread, rye, whole meal - 41–55	Watermelon, raw - 72–80
Bread, rye, whole meal - 62–66	
Bread, sunflower and barley - 57	
Bread, wheat, refined - 77–80	
Bread, wheat, white - 59–69	
Bread, wheat, white, high-fiber - 65–69	
Bread, wheat, whole - 71–87	
Bread, wheat, whole meal - 67	
Bread, wheat, whole meal - 64–69	
Bread, white - 55	
Bread, white, gluten-free - 71-80	
Bread, whole meal - 53	
Croissant – 67	

http://www.all4naturalhealth.com/glycemic-index-listing.html

Glycemic Load

This is important as eating too much sugar or carbohydrates may lead to dis-eases like cancer. The medical establishment does not make these links widely known to the uneducated populace. Perhaps it has to do with their profit margin. The more you know, the less likelihood of you getting sick. I observed lack of knowledge the other day while waiting for my car which was being diagnosed at the local service station. This station is directly across the street from a middle school. Teen after teen came in to purchase their... breakfast? They purchased sugar drinks, candy bars, bags of chips and crackers. So, at 7:00 in the morning, they were eating sugar, salt, hydrogenated oils - the five whites, – for breakfast. I was appalled, but this is the norm for many American youth. While visiting Ghana a few years ago I saw a flood of junk food being sold on the streets to another unknowing populace. I later found out that much of this food is being imported from China and of course Europe. The unknowledgeable eating their way to early disease and destruction or dependence on big pharmacies for a large portion of their lives.

Dr. Otto Warburg, Nobel Prize winner, established very clearly the direct relationship between sugar and cancer. When you normalize your sugar level, the reduction of your glycemic load will improve your health and lower your risk to cancer and other disorders. Be aware that the sugars and carbohydrates that you eat which convert to sugar can kill you. My mother, may she rest in power, loved sugar; she made sweets all the time for her biological and church family. Her desserts were out of this world good, but not good for you. She developed diabetes. Later in life she developed cancer in the bone. But you could not tell her it had to do with her eating. Also when we don't get enough love and affection, we might turn to sugar, emotional eating. People of color live in a hostile world, hated by many for the melanin in our skin as well as other gifts bestowed upon us by the Creator. It is not a surprise that diabetes runs rampant in our communities. But we can and must turn this around. If you know better you must do better. Each one, teach one.

Diets high in sugar can also cause hypertension, obesity, high cholesterol and other lipids, heart disease, kidney disease, female infertility and neuro (brain) issues. Sugar blues are for real for real. This white sugar thang is bad news 360. Please note too much sugar, even the natural kind, is bad news. It is addictive; your body starts wanting it like a drug. Pay attention and monitor your glycemic load. Seek help if you must. Sugar will jam you up! The jam session will be in the doctor's office, you getting your prescriptions, which all have side effects. Then the jam session will be in the laboratory, you getting tested and possibly radiated at the same time! If you still don't wake up the jam session will be you hooked up to some machine for the rest of your life for many days a week. Then it's off to party in the surgical theater where you could lose a toe or a limb. Are we jamming? Or jammed? Skip the jelly rolls.

Then of course the impact it has on the destruction of your teeth. Don't believe me? Take one of your favorite sugary drinks and drop a tooth in it for a week. Sugar will decay it and dissolve it in no time! Word to the wise should be sufficient. In the old days we got sweets once in a while, not more than one a week. The old people knew what was up and they didn't need no PhD.

Gluten = WORBs

Many people have a problem with the **WORBs**. So this information is included so you can make an educated decision. Now I know you are wondering what in the world is the WORBs. Simple - it is a way to help you remember what has Gluten in it W – Wheat, O – Oats (has gluten if processed with other gluten foods), R – Rye, and B – Barley: the WORBs

You will see entire sections in some supermarkets that are dedicated to gluten free products or WORBs free. WORBs give many folks digestive problems. The human body is amazing as demonstrated by the clearing up of health problems when certain foods are eliminated. Even if they don't give you a problem it is probably a good idea not to veg out on them. If you have a healing challenge, weight issue or simply want to keep your glow on and look young and vibrant - skip the WORBs.

While we are on the topic of grains, many food educators suggest that eating any grain is a waste of time, as they are nutrient void. (If you want to do more research on that topic check the writings of Doug Graham, DC, *Grain Damage* and George A. Malkamus, *God's Way to Ultimate Health)*. I think eating sprouted grain is the best option. You should not eat even a spoonful of flour, that is not found in nature (white flour, bleached flour, enriched flour). Hence the debate on grains, I have observed that a diet heavy in grains, pasta, cereal makes me fat. Others experience a hung over feeling or a sedated feeling. Some compare flour to glue. Nowadays many people are using ground nuts, almond and coconut instead of flour from grains. So you have options, now that you know that eating all that flour is not in your highest interest.

Be your own scientist, experiment on yourself, go without it for a period and see how you look and feel. Queen Afua has always stated that the factory is the corporate kitchen and not a healing kitchen. Spend more time in your own healing kitchen preparing food from your garden, food coop, farmer's market, organic or health food store. If you don't have much space, learn to sprout right in the kitchen and make a container garden. Where there is a will to be healthy, there is a way.

Some general information about protein from vegan sources

There is a huge misconception that vegetarians can't get enough protein. National and international recommendations for protein intake are based on animal sources of protein such as meat, cow's milk and eggs. Plant proteins get a bad rap because they are sometimes less digestible due to differences in the nature of the protein and the presence of other factors such as fiber. Nevertheless, dietary studies show the adequacy of plant foods as sole sources of protein as does the experience of healthy vegans of all ages.

On average, fruits have about 5% of their calories from protein. Vegetables have from 20-50% of their calories from protein. Sprouted seeds, beans, and grains contain from 10-25% of their calories from protein. Numerous scientific studies have shown the daily need for protein to be about 25-35 grams per day. So if you ate 2,000 calories per day, and ate raw plant foods that had an average of 10% of their calories from protein, you would get 200 calories worth of protein, or 50 grams. This is more than adequate to support optimal well-being. (Yet another reason to eat a high live diet).

The misguided idea that plant proteins are not "complete" is based on studies done on rats in the 1940's. This false conclusion was drawn before we discovered the body's protein recycling mechanism and its ability to "complete" any amino acid mix from our body's amino acid pool, no matter what the amino acid composition of a meal consumed. This false idea is still perpetuated by the meat and dairy industries.

Protein is made in the human body out of individual amino acids. Food is broken into individual amino acids and then reassembles the proteins it requires. It used to be believed that all amino acids must be eaten at the same time to form complete proteins. We now know that incomplete proteins can be stored in the body for many days to be combined with other incomplete proteins. As long as all essential amino acids are in the diet, it does not matter if the proteins are complete or incomplete.

The main protein foods in a vegan diet are the pulses (peas, beans and lentils), nuts, seeds and grains. As the average protein level in pulses is 27% of calories; in nuts and seeds 13%; and in grains 12%, it is easy to see that plant foods can supply the recommended amount of protein as long as the energy requirements are met.

There is much information on vegan athletes and how they manage protein. I used a protein supplement from Young Living for myself and my daughter when she was a child just to make sure we were getting our daily needs met. To this day, I still use this non-soy protein powder in my morning juice or smoothie. For those who would like to order it, it is called **Power Meal.** (Ordering info in back of book).

Ani Bere

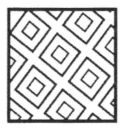

Perseverance and Diligence

Eat Your Greens & Redeem your Power
Green Leafy Vegetables

"Look younger, feel younger – drink your greens" As you transition to a plant based diet, please consider the following. Some animals, including primates who are primarily vegetarians, consume large quantities of green leaves. Some raw foodists advocate that humans may need to consume 40% of green leaves in their diet which is nutritionally beneficial.

One cannot argue with the benefits of a diet high in leafy greens, the darker the better! However, to consume 40% of one's calories on a daily basis, might be challenging. The uncooked greens are considered optimal because all the enzymes, vitamins, minerals and amino acids would be held intact and not destroyed or reduced due to the activity of heat. Some would say the sun has already cooked our food, so why do we need to cook it again? One way to infuse more greens into your diet is eating them in a blended form, where they are pre-digested. You can also prepare them in the form of soups, smoothies and puddings. If you choose to include the blended foods as a part of your diet, then be sure to not skip the chewing process. At this point you are going to need to invest in a hefty blender. I like Vita Mixer, they are very strong with lengthy warranties. D. Do your research, there are many to choose from.

Of course salads and green wraps are additional options. Wrapping your food in a green cabbage or collard leaf, gives you another alternative to starchy taco, tortilla and grain dishes. You could even use Nori (seaweed) paper. Just make sure it does not come from Japan. I don't want you eating radiated food sources! My suggestion is not to use the same leaf, in your smoothie, but to change it every 4/5 days. Overuse of one type of leaf, will begin to minimize the positive effects that this process has on the body. You could work with spinach, then kale, next dandelion or Swiss chard. Edible weeds such as chicory, rose-hips, nasturtium, watercress, plantain, sour grass, purslane, dandelion, lambs quarters, Jerusalem Artichoke, red clover, mint, parsley, chives, or comfrey can also be used.

When first starting do not overuse the stems as they may have a very strong taste; However be sure to use the stems if your body is very toxic with improper living and eating. Take it slow. Some of these weeds may need to be juiced then added to the blended drink. Test them out, observe your body's reaction and do what is best for you at the time.

Dandelion exceeds all edible greens in vitamin A content by at least 4X. Purslane tops all the greens except parsley, in organic iron content. Sorrell contains 3X more vitamin C than lemons. The grasses exceed even the common weeds in nutrition value. Word to the wise, cold foods on a prolonged basis are not in the best interest of the body. They will have a negative impact on your digestive system. (This goes for ice cubes and ice cream.) Therefore, cold smoothies are a no-no, not in your best interest if you cherish your health. Room temperature is optimal. Knock the chill off of them by placing the container in some warm water for a few minutes or in the oven on low for a minute.

If you don't have time for smoothies on a regular basis, then make it the night before or in a real crunch, take some green supplements! Still, get your greens in every day in every way. See the section on recipes for the green smoothie combination. It's the queen of smoothie. Have some fun, you just have to get over the idea that it is green. They taste really good.

Wheatgrass Juice

I have lived on wheatgrass for a period of time as a part of a detoxification plan which included 100% raw or living foods. Whenever there is illness amongst my family or friends I always recommend wheatgrass juice. I also feel that a maintenance plan would include weekly or monthly infusions of wheat grass juice. I might also add that is not one of my favorite juices, but the benefits to health are outstanding, including its ability to prevent Free Radical and lipofuscin pigments from accumulating and doing their damage. A healthy body requires healthy blood; after all it is the blood that carries the nutrients to every part of the body. In the book *Chlorophyll Magic from Living Plant Life,* Dr. Jensen recounts how he was able to increase red blood count by having the patient soak in chlorophyll-water baths. He also noted that this process occurs even faster when the patient drinks green juices, blended drinks and wheat grass juice. See the *Wheatgrass Book* by Dr. Ann Wigmore for more information on wheatgrass and Living foods.

These are some of the benefits I experienced:

- ❖ Clear mind
- ❖ Greater memory power
- ❖ Exceptional energy
- ❖ Weight loss
- ❖ Clear eyes
- ❖ Bright aura/glow
- ❖ Rejuvenating
- ❖ Colon cleanser

Benefits/observations from Ann Wigmore, ND:

70% chlorophyll

Chlorophyll is light energy

It is highly sterile solution

Can be digested in minutes using very little energy

Science has proven that chlorophyll arrest the growth and development of unfriendly bacteria

Wheatgrass rebuilds the bloodstream

Restores the sex hormones

Liquid chlorophyll aids in removing drug deposits from the body

Chlorophyll neutralizes toxins in the body.

Chlorophyll improves blood sugar problems

Wheatgrass juice assists with high blood pressure

Ani Bere

Nutrient Milligrams per pound

Chlorophyll	5000mg
Choline	4000mg
Vitamin C	2000mg
Vitamin A	360mg
Vitamin E	120mg
Vitamin F	120mg
Vitamin K	120mg
Niacin	120mg
Vitamin B-2	24
Vitamin B-1	12
Pantothenic Acid	8mg
Vitamin B-6	4mg

Where to purchase??

Call your local Health Food/Co-op and inquire if they carry the wheatgrass growing in trays. Sometimes it is sold already cut, I prefer it still growing. Some people learn to grow their own at home. If the store does not carry it on a regular basis, see if they will special order it for you. You will eventually need to invest in a wheatgrass juicer.

When you can't make fresh green drinks or juices, then by all means supplement with a green powder product. Eat greens or a green supplement on a daily basis.

OUR JOURNEY: RED, BLACK, GREEN AND VEGAN

Denkyem

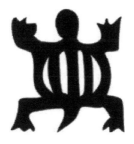

Adaptability

Tidbits to Keep you Healthy!

Jump start your vitality with sprouts!

Sprouts release mucous-forming inhibitors. They are easily digested into concentrated proteins providing balanced high energy nourishment that is primarily alkaline forming. Simply put sprouts are a super food that you should consider adding to your salads, juices and green smoothies, fruit smoothies, sandwiches or green wraps.

If you are on a road trip and have difficulty finding a place to eat, buy some sprouts from the supermarket, add some lemon or salad dressing and start munching. You will feel added energy in a short time. Chew well, until they are liquefied in your mouth.

Sprouts can also be grown at home at little expense or effort. They are an acquired taste.

411 on Water

Understand that our bodies are primarily water—some say 60-70%. So it is important to drink water. The more active you are the more water you need. Our needs vary, so observing your urine is critical. The color of urine should be light yellow. If the smell is intense, you need more water. My mother wit indicates that if your body odor is strong you need more water and you need to detox. Women your lady parts should smell like a flower nice and sweet. If it smells like fish, you have a problem that needs time and attention. Water will help. Men if your man parts are *funky wonky* along with your armpits and your feet, OMG, take a bath and drink more water!

At the **Healing Tree Detox Spa** we have an herbal steam treatment that will also address genital funk. Funk is for music, not your body

Additional signs that you need to increase your water intake are the following:

❖ Fatigue and/or mood swings

❖ Hunger even though you've recently eaten

❖ Back or joint ache

❖ Dull, dry skin and/or pronounced wrinkles

❖ Infrequent urination; dark, concentrated urine, and/or constipation

Signs of chronic dehydration which include the following:

❖ Digestive disturbances: heartburn, gallstones and constipation

❖ Confusion/anxiety

❖ Urinary tract infections

❖ Premature aging

❖ High cholesterol

Overeating can be a sign of dehydration. If you keep eating, then your body probably needs more water not food. Twenty percent of water in the body is derived from fruits and vegetables. So it's good you're going vegan. Consider purchasing a home water filtration system. Drinking water out of plastic is not healthy for you or the environment. Soft plastic may leach chemicals into your water. These chemicals may cause men to be less masculine. Caution is critical with foods and water packaged in soft plastics.

Water stored in severe cold or severe heat, may also be contaminated by the chemicals in the plastic as it is frozen or heated and released into the water. Do not leave bottled water in your car planning to drink it later on.

Unfiltered tap water does not promote health. Drinking juice does not replace the bodies need for water. (The elders would often squeeze a fresh lemon in their water, especially in the morning to break up waste and mucous. This helps detox the body). Most of USA tap water is recycled sewage water. Can you imagine? This is almost as insane as feeding livestock its own flesh and then wondering where mad cow syndrome came from. At any rate you will want to invest in a home water filtration system that will clean and alkalize your water. In my modest home, I have a whole house water filtration unit. Nothing fancy, think I purchased it at Home Depot. I like it because it takes out fluoride and other substances. However, the filter must be changed frequently. I wanted to have fluoride removed so when I am in the bath tub or the Jacuzzi, I am not sitting in a chemical soup which may dumb me down and calcify the pineal gland, aka, third eye. (This is the organ which assists in visions and knowing). I also don't buy toothpaste that has fluoride.

You might want to check out the Nikken water purifier for the counter top for food and drinking. I like Nikken as you can create a stream of income with their products. Their products are top shelf. But do your research on water; you will be amazed at the information and all the products available. If you can afford the $4000 dollar model then get it for yourself and family. An ounce of prevention is worth a pound of cure.

Adding a little chlorophyll or fresh lemon to your water will help to keep it alkaline.

Drinking pure coconut water without added sugars or chemicals is a great substitute for water. When in the tropics, I just drink the divine waters of the coconut. I drink it now as much as I can afford, especially during detox and fasting cycles. Yum yum! When I am on the road and need a drink, it's not juice I look for but coconut water. When I lived in Ghana there was a brother who lived near me who was a fruitarian. He was also an athlete, his muscles rippled. (Yes, he was fine.) He had coconuts delivered to his residence several times a week. He used them for drinking and making fruit salads with the juice and the meat. This was in the 70's. Brother was ahead of the game.

Conscious Power Eating

Sit down and relax when you eat, digestion belongs to the Queen, the parasympathetic system. That system is about rest, relaxation and healing. I call the system female compared to the circulatory system which is more male due to that heart, which is always on duty. The parasympathetic system has no pump. So the nature of it is a little slower, chilled out—like females are traditionally. So when you eat, you are under the domain of the Parasympathetic Goddess/Queen. Slow down, relax, enjoy the moment. Concentrate on chewing your food 50x-100x before swallowing it. I know you are like "WHAT??" but hang with me. This allows the enzymes in the mouth to mix with the food which helps the digestive process. You could also try putting your eating utensils down while chewing.

This method will help you not to over eat as well as lose weight. In this silence you can give thanks, grace and gratitude to the elements who gave so you could have this food to nourish your body. Give thanks to the air, water, soil, sun, wind, humans and the Creator for all that took part in growing this food that is now nourishing your body. After you have given thanks count mentally, silently how many times you are chewing each mouthful of food. Eat in silence or talk after the meal is completed or in between courses. Let your meal mates know in advance so they won't feel any way about it. You will find what works for you. This technique has helped many who found themselves imprisoned/detained or without the means to buy or grow food. Your body will get more out of less food when you consciously chew it thoroughly. Some say when we skip pre-digestion by not chewing and thoroughly masticating our food, we overeat.

Supplementing with Vitamins

I am a person who never liked to take drugs or even vitamins. As an adult I did not like going to the western trained doctor. I would go for the diagnosis then work my natural knowledge to heal and return to balance. I am sure this is due to my great grandmother who was an herbalist. However, I was taught by some more seasoned vegans, that American soil lacks many minerals due to lack of rotation farming methods and the chemicals that are constantly used to assault the soil in the form of herbicides, pesticides and now GMO farming standards. To be healthy one must grow one's own food and/or supplement with vitamins and minerals. I do not recommend that you purchase these from a drug store. Buy the highest quality you can afford. Often your holistic practitioner will order them for you from a quality supplier. The ones to consider on a daily basis are as follows:

❖   liquid iron
❖   liquid calcium/magnesium
❖   multiple vitamin for men, women and children
❖   B vitamin complex
❖   Moringa or Spirulina
❖   Kelp
❖   vitamin C
❖   vitamin D

Denkyem

I especially suggest a supplement for children. Hopefully, they are making this journey with you. My own daughter had liquid calcium, iron and a protein shake/smoothie five days a week when she was under my tutelage. She has great teeth, skin intellect, and fabulous spirit!

If you just can't get with the supplement regimen, the following list is adapted from Sistah Zakhah's book *The Joy of Living Live, A Raw Food Journey* published by Communicators Press. I highly recommend her work. She chooses to supplement with foods, rather than vitamins. Choose the method that works for you and your family.

- ❖ Blackstrap Molasses
- ❖ Sesame Seeds
- ❖ Kelp
- ❖ Brewer's yeast
- ❖ Fresh parsley
- ❖ Fenugreek
- ❖ Wheat germ

These items are recommended to be taken on a daily basis for those 10 years and older. I would add nut milk and green smoothies to this list. Recipes for nut milk are included in the last chapter.

I have recently discovered Juice Plus. It is a whole food supplement. Please check it out, I really like it. zatiti.juiceplus.com I think it is excellent for travel, emergencies and as a regular nutritional support. The reseach is very impressive for adults and children. Think of it as juice without juicing. The crewables are crazy good!

Aya

Endurance and Resourcefulness

Staying On Top

Remember the earlier chart on the different types of plant eaters (on page 40)? You will have discovered that a Living/raw food diet is at the top of the chart. Some of my readers will want to transition to that type diet if not fully, then to a high percentage. We call it **high live**. I transition to a fruitarian diet from May to October, as I currently live in a cold region.

This is an exceptional way to see, how living on fruits will benefit your chi/energy. I lose weight/waste, have a better glow and more energy. I detox more while on the diet, naturally and intentionally. Some of my readers may choose a Raw, Live or High Live path. For your education,I have included items needed for the Live-food kitchen.

Items for a Living Food Kitchen

1. Coffee grinder for grinding nuts and seeds
2. Cutting mats/boards
3. Food dehydrator preferably an Excalibur
4. Food processor

5. High Speed blender preferably a Vitamix

6. Juicers for citrus fruits and vegetable/fruits and wheat grass

7. Knives

8. Mandoline Slicer

These are less critical, but still quite useful:

    a. Garlic press

    b. Rubber spatula

    c. Salad spinner

    d. Measure tools

    e. Wire strainers

    f. Glass jars for juices

    g. Sprouting containers/kits are available

    h. Pineapple cutter

    i. Weight scale

Some of these items can be a little pricey but if they are good quality, you won't have to replace them for many years. Thrift stores are also a possible way to acquire any one of these items until you can get a new one. Check on eBay and Craigslist for items that are being recycled. Give your family a wish list for your birthday or Kwanzaa. Also, consider purchasing lower end products at the beginning of your journey. Big Lots and Bed, Bath and Beyond are two stores that may have what you need.

Aya

Food Combining

Food combining is a difficult topic for me to address, perhaps because I'm always breaking the "rules". I also look at some of the traditional foods from my African ancestry and see that these rules were not always adhered too. It just makes me wonder if our production of enzymes and digestive processes are the same as others. **Most health research is normed on Caucasians and not on people of Nubian/Afrikan descent**. For example rice is a staple in most West African countries, and it is eaten with beans and other proteins as well as peanuts. Well according to the food combining rules this is a no-no?? Also in Ghana, fufu, a daily staple food is made of plantains and cassava, a fruit and a starch – another supposed no-no. We don't have to look to Africa, look at red beans and corn bread. This is an area needing research. Nevertheless, I thought I would pass on the information.

I have recently learned that a protruding stomach may be due to poor food combining. Now that peaks my interest, a waist line of note, yeah ok, that would be dope! I'll food combine. Place this chart in your healing kitchen **and refer to it as you learn to be an educated veggie.** Just do your best. Also pay attention to what gives you gas, makes you belch or just doesn't digest well. Then look at what you eat and what you eat with it. Tweak your eating habits to fit your person. Pick your health providers brains as well.

These are the basics:
- Proteins should be eaten with non starch vegetables
- Starchy vegetables should be eaten with non starch vegetables and greens
- Eat melons alone or leave them alone
- Consume liquids by themselves

- Eat fruits in the morning and within their tribe/family
- Eat Citrus fruit together:
  - a. Oranges
  - b. Lemons
  - c. Grapefruit
  - d. Limes
  - e. Pomegranates

- Eat Sub acids fruits together
  - a. Sweet cherry
  - b. Fig
  - c. Grape
  - d. Apple
  - e. Apricot
  - f. Mango
  - g. Papaya
  - h. pear

  Eat Sweet fruits together
  - a. Raisin
  - b. Persimmon
  - c. Bananas
  - d. Dried fruits

- Though it is best to eat them in their category (family), sub acid Fruits can be eaten with acid or sweet fruits, this is considered a fair combination.

(The live foodist indicates that fruits can be eaten with green leafy vegetables, but I generally only use sub acid and the berry family).

This is information that you will want to incorporate as you develop a sound footing on this path. I am still working on this after being a veggie for 30 plus years. So do your best, but don't trip on it. However if you notice that certain combinations don't agree with your digestive process, in that you have monster gas, bloating diarrhea or constipation, then you should not ignore your symptoms - you should change and not eat that combination. Some food advocates suggest eating one food at a time, this does not over tax the system and makes digestion a breeze.

Another difficulty with food combining is that many of the charts contradict each other, or offer exceptions to the rules. So I suggest you use them as generalities and not as the law. Pay attention to your temple and how it responds to the eating of certain foods.

Know that different foods require different digestive fluids to do the work in breaking down the food. You do not want to wash these fluids away by drinking during eating or immediately after.

FOOD COMBINING CHART

STARCHY VEGGIES NON STARCHY VEGGIES GRAINS SWEET FRUITS SUB ACID FRUITS ACID FRUITS MELONS

PROTEIN

(ONLY COMBINE WHEN CIRCLES DIRECTLY
TOUCH FOR OPTIMAL DIGESTION)

STARCHY VEGGIES	NON STARCH VEGGIES	GRAINS	PROTEIN	SWEET FRUITS	SUB ACID FRUITS	ACID FRUITS	MELONS
ARTICHOKES	ASPARAGUS	AMARANTH	MEAT	BANANA	SWEET CHERRIES	GRAPEFRUIT	CANTALOUPE
BEETS	BELL PEPPER	BUCKWHEAT	FISH	DATES	APPLES	ORANGE	HONEYDEW
CARROTS	BROCCOLI	QUINOA	AVOCADO	FIGS	BERRIES	LEMON	WATERMELON
CORN	BRUSSEL SPROUTS	MILLET	BEANS	DRIED FRUITS	APRICOT	LIME	MUSKMELON
JICAMA	CABBAGE	OATS	NUTS	PERSIMMON	PAPAYA	PINEAPPLE	CRENSHAW
PEAS	CELERY	RICE	SEEDS	PRUNES	PEAR	POMEGRANATE	
POTATOES	CHARD	SPELT		GRAPES	MANGO	CRANBERRIES	
PUMPKIN	COLLARDS	WHEAT			PEACHES	SOUR APPLE	
SQUASH	CUCUMBER	FLOUR			PLUMS	STRAWBERRIES	
YAMS	GARLIC						
	GREEN BEANS						
	KALE						
	LEEK						
	LETTUCE						
	ONIONS						
	PARSLEY						
	RHUBARB						
	SPINACH						
	SUMMER SQUASH						
	TOMATOES						
	TURNIP						
	ZUCCHINI						

snapandsprouts.com

110

Fasting Options

You may want to read and consider this section after you have made sound improvements on the step pyramid that begins on page 44. But if you have a serious health challenge then generally it is advisable to detox your toxic load asap. Fasting will help you to do this. Most animals stop eating when ill. Humans have learned to override this wisdom. The following edited contribution was submitted by my long-time friend **Mark Blake**, who is a disciplined raw foodist and wellness coach. You can find him on facebook.

Here is a list of some fasting options. Take time to consider what's ideal for you and remember that it's not something we're forcing on ourselves; it's something we're giving ourselves....

A quick note: blending fruits and vegetables is different than juicing – juicing is extracting the pulp (fiber). With blending you get to assimilate your food better and give the body a rest from your regular diet. With juicing, you are eliminating a major portion of the digestive cycle and freeing up a lot of body energy that can be used to detox and repair. You also do not experience the daily hunger after the 2nd day or so... both have great benefits.

I recommend each person do some research and investigate and see what resonates with you.

(1) The Master Cleanse: This is a great cleanse, and it is doable even for those without blenders, juicers and other utensils. 4oz grade B maple syrup/4ounces fresh squeezed lemon juice/

32oz spring, filtered or distilled water. Mix all together with about 1/8 tsp cayenne pepper. You'll probably drink 2 or 3 of these batches a day. It's important that we each put effort into our process. Use fresh squeezed organic lemons for the lemon juice and not commercial pasteurized (heated) juice. In addition, it's best to not put the cayenne pepper in until you are ready to have your drink. Those w/ blood sugar imbalances like diabetes or hypoglycemia may find this cleanse challenging because of the high sugar content in the maple syrup (use grade b dark maple syrup). If you do choose this method and have blood sugar issues I would take either a tablespoon full of raw hemp protein powder, or a teaspoon full of spirulina w/ each serving you have. I suggest you do a Smooth Move, or senna tea occasionally to help get the toxins out. Sea salt water flush (SWF) is mention, although I do not recommend this every day.

(2) Water fast: This can be challenging and I usually only recommend this to people who have done previous fasting, are in good health, or have certain life threatening situations to be cured from. The water fast requires you to do a lot of resting. Attempting to be very active is counter to this type of fast. Drink either spring water, filtered water, or fresh water from the source. A nice 30 minute walk twice a day is helpful, as well as deep breathing exercises, and some mild yoga. Remember that you will not be replacing any nutrients, so do not make high demands on the body's energy level. During this fast colonics, or water enemas can be helpful to get rid of impacted waste (the sea salt water flush like in the master cleanse will change the nature of this fast and prevent you from going into the fasting mode, so it's not recommended).

(3) Green juice fast: for those who have a good juicer like the champion, green star, or other slow turning juicers that juice

leafy green vegetables well. It consists of drinking just green juices from fruits (like cucumber and zucchini), and vegetables (like kale, collards, celery, chard, etc.) and juicing in a lemon w/ each 48oz batch will help take the pungent taste away from the dark green juices. Drink as much as you have thirst for, and in addition drink herbal teas (unsweetened) and water. This is great for those w/ blood sugar imbalances. It is also good for those who struggle to keep weight on, because the high minerals will minimize loss of muscle mass and mainly give you a loss in fats, and waste. This is my favorite fast.

(4) Coconut water fast: This consists of drinking fresh young coconut water every day, as much as you have thirst for. Many of the ethnic markets will have young Thai coconuts, and some areas of the country have organic coconuts. You can do a google search for instructions on opening them. Expect to do at least 4 -5 a day, and maybe even more. Many health food stores also carry coconut water in the one liter container. This can be a substitute, although because it is pasteurized it does not have the life energy so I would add 1 full T of spirulina to each liter container. Expect to go through 3-4 or more liters per day.... This keeps you very hydrated. You will also be consuming filtered or spring water, and if you desire some herbal teas. Garden of Life also makes a nice raw green powder which is great for extra minerals instead of just spirulina, especially if you're working out.

(5) Watermelon fast: This is a very cleansing fast that keeps your body nice and cool and hydrated in a hot climate. Use only watermelons w/ seeds in it, preferably organic and/or locally grown. Eat as much as you like, or blend it up into a smoothie, including the seeds. The seeds will help with digestion and parasites. Those with blood sugar imbalances may wish to blend it with protein powder (hemp or flax), or a green powder (like

spirulina, etc.). Use this method when in season.

(6) All raw fast: consists of all raw organic fruits, sprouts, and vegetables (no nuts, seeds, dehydrated or sun-dried foods). Eat as much as you like, although you may find eating small meals throughout the day easier for the body to digest and break-down. For those w/ colon challenges, do some green smoothies to get your greens down (www.rawfoods.com has some great free recipes).

(7) Fruit fast: this is a very cleansing fast and great for those with digestive disorders. It is also good for those not yet ready for a liquid fast. Consume only organic fruits, preferably locally grown. Diabetics and others with hypoglycemic concerns should proceed with caution and stay away from the super sweet fruits, bananas, any dried fruits, and mangoes. Use only fruits with seeds. Apples help regulate blood sugar. Pears do not affect blood sugar levels like other fruit. Anything in the cherry/berry family is great. Remember to have plenty of the non-sweet fruits (avocados, tomatoes, eggplants, olives, squash, etc) You may find that you are drinking less water which is OK, since you will be consuming plenty of water that is filtered through the fibers of the fruit.

It's important that you move your body every day. A brisk walk 2x a day, some yoga, calisthenics etc. are great and don't have to be done to the point of exhaustion. Keep in mind the lymph glands eliminate toxins but don't have a pump like the heart so they need movement to assist in getting stuff out. I recom-mend getting a rebounder and doing about 20 minutes of light jumping in the morning on the rebounder, or as much as you can without overextending yourself. This will help keep the skin tight as you lose the pounds. If you're not exercising you'll find many of the toxins that are released go right back into the blood stream.

You may have days when you're tired or eliminating toxins at a rapid rate. Don't fight that period, take the needed rest or breathe, meditate; expect. It is a great idea for us to take pictures on our first day, and compare them to our final day. Cut down on the TV/radio, internet, negative people etc.

Ananse Ntontan

Ananse NtontanAnanse Ntontan

RECIPES

I cook like an artist. My kitchen time is my time to create. This section may drive some of you krazy. Some of the recipes are without measurement because I work with my creativity in the kitchen, not my left brain. That said, these recipes are not really recipes but general guides to help you create your own delicious entrees.

I come from a line of Nubian women who for the most part do not measure, and yet the food comes out great! And if it doesn't, we just try it again, tweaking our spices, quantities and other ingredients.

When preparing veggies, always use color and texture. This will keep your dishes exciting and seductive. A little red, a little green, a little purple, to spice up the energy in a dish. Keep a grater and a food processor on hand to help give you the color you need in a dish. If cooking, remember to add the most delicate plant last, so as not to overcook it and spoil its beautiful color...not to mention killing the nutrients. Some of my dishes are merely warmed salads. I cook them very little. This will help you get the needed nutrients from food rather than eating empty calories. This process is called *al dente*.

Keep trying to make your food a little better each time you prepare it. For example, I can prepare carob dishes in countless ways, because I keep changing and/or embellishing the base recipe. So have fun as you create in your healing room. Never prepare food when you are angry or in other ill spirits. Your food, like a canvas, will reflect the energy of your dominant mood.

I have also added some of my favorite chefs in this section, many who do measure. Sample the work of Chef Elaine, Chef Heru, Chef Kunti, Chef Linda, Chef Sheeba, Chef Akua and Chef Tomi from UK by way of Nigeria! Our recipes are organized into Breakfast Ideas and anytime Smoothies, Living Food Entrees, Cooked Entrees and A La Carte, Not Meats and Tasty Treats.

BREAK – FAST Ideas & ANYTIME SMOOTHIES

Fruit Soup

This is basically a fruit smoothie that you serve in a bowl with a pretty garnish!

Thicken it with ground seeds, soaked nuts or dried fruit. I like flax, egbono or sesame seeds. Place in a warmed oven/dehydrator for a minute to knock the chill off. Serve!

Fruit Stew

This is a thick fruit soup with large pieces of fruit in the liquid.

Ananse Ntontan

Water Melon Stew

Chop up the desired amount of watermelon and other melons
Blend some in the blender. Set others aside.
Add ground flax seed to watermelon juice.
Pour into serving dishes.
Add chopped cantaloupe, honey dew or other melons of your choice.
Garnish with a sprig of parsley.

Strawberry Stew

Organic Strawberries, blackberries or blueberries
Organic yellow apple
Coconut water or coconut milk
Make your smoothie with strawberries, apples and coconut liquid of your choice
Save some whole pieces for the stew
Pour your strawberry smoothie into bowls
Add your chopped apples and whole berries
Garnish!
Stew can always be thickened with flax seed or sesame seeds or protein powder.

Nut Milk

1 cup organic raw almonds soaked for 24 hours
Store in refrigerator while soaking
Use filtered water

Peel all the brown skin off the nuts
Place in them to the Vita Mixer or Blender

Add 2 cups of water and blend
Add a drop of organic vanilla
Add Stevia to sweeten
Blend, strain and keep in the refrigerator to use in all recipes that require milk.

If you want to drink it, add a piece of fruit to sweeten

Strain, but do not toss out the nut meat, use in veggie burgers, top of a salad or dehydrated recipes.

Raw Oatmeal

Organic whole oats
1 or 2 T organic raisins
Soaked walnuts
Sprinkle cinnamon
Stevia (optional)/raw sugar
Coconut milk or any vegan milk

Soak oatmeal in nut milk until desired consistency is reached, 5-15 minutes. Add the other ingredients to your liking. Place in slightly warm oven to warm.

Ananse Ntontan

Green Smoothies

great in the morning   ~   variations are limitless

3/6 Large leaves Kale,
1 organic apple &
2 slices of fresh organic pineapple,
Filtered water

Organic blueberries (or any berry)
Banana
Apple
Coconut water or milk

2 collard green leaves, cut out stem
1 apple
2 slices of fresh organic pineapple

Coconut or almond milk
Cinnamon
1-4 cups of baby spinach
1 organic apple cored
1 cup of papaya (non GMO)
1-2 cups filtered water

Cantaloupe, Honeydew and/or Watermelon (seeded)
Coconut water

Beet Greens
Mango Ripe and sliced
Some green sprouts
1-2 cups water
small amount of watercress

Cucumber
Apple
Mango
Coconut water

Add healthy supplements to taste, including: Rice protein powder, chia seed, moringa, spirulina, ground flax seed, ground sesame seeds, etc.

Cinnamon, ginger, cardamom, fresh garlic, even seeded jalapeño makes smoothies more interesting. Play, create and discover!

Ananse Ntontan

Master Green Smoothie

Organic Greens, apples and organic berries, sprouts, filtered water.

Greens are a very important element of our diet, try to drink 8-64 oz of blended greens daily, and slowly increasing the oz each week. Try it, you will be amazed! Please don't forget to add sprouts and wild weeds, and fresh herbs and supplements to your smoothie once you get used to the daily green drill. Consider including spirulina, moringa and protein non-soy powder like Power Meal from Youngliving.com. This is in addition to the fresh leafy greens.

Use the glycemic index and the food combining chart when you make your smoothies. In the long run your digestive system will thank you, however some nutritional detours every once in a while are forgivable. Some digestive systems cannot tolerate transgressions.

The greens will keep your system in top condition with frequent trips to the bathroom. So when nature calls you better answer promptly. The regular drinking of green may increase the transit time of your bowels. In other words, they start to move fast, so you will need to get to steppin' when nature gives you the signal.

Use fruit in your smoothies in the beginning and over time begin to make the smoothies with less and less fruit. In the beginning the body will require a larger quantity; in time the needs will be less, but a more concentrated green drink.

Smoothie Combinations

1. Fresh or frozen organic Strawberries
2. Apples, water, apple juice or coconut milk
3. Water or organic apple juice
4. Pineapple, Apple ginger root, water
5. Cranberry, apple, raspberry, water or apple juice
6. Frozen organic berries with banana, and nut milk or water
7. Pears, bananas and coconut milk or water
8. Kiwi, apples, berries of your choice, water, nut milk or apple organic juice
9. Mango, apple banana with water or nut milk

Do not overuse mango or any really sweet fruit in smoothies, or you may get cavities or diabetes.

Make your own combination, later add your supplements and protein powder like Power Meal, from youngliving.com.

LIVING FOOD ENTREES

Cauliflower "Potato" Salad

1 head of fresh organic Cauliflower
1 cup tomatoes
2-3 T Veganaise (vegan mayo, found in refrigeration section)
1 grated carrot
¼ c red onions
¾ c green onions diced
½ c diced celery
chopped parsley
2t **diluted** Braggs Liquid Aminos (or the non- soy one made with coconut)
garlic powder to taste
dash of red pepper (optional)
dash of cumin (optional)
organic dill pickle relish

Break up head of cauliflower into small bite-sized pieces.
Add the other ingredients and mix into a beautiful salad.

Carrot Tuna

Chop in large pieces 5 organic carrots
Process in food processor to desired texture
Add 2T olive oil
Add red onions, green onions tops, tomatoes diced,
½ c chopped parsley for additional color
½ c sprouts
2t garlic powder to taste
2t kelp powder (optional)

Use Bragg's Liquid Aminos or Coconut Aminos to taste
Makes about 6 servings

Collard or any Leafy Green Salad

2 bunches of Organic Collard or Kale Greens
Juice of fresh organic lemon & essential oil of lemon
3T Extra Virgin cold pressed Olive oil
3 cloves of Fresh garlic minced
¼ c red onions diced
¼ c green sprouts
½ c diced tomatoes

- Wash greens 3x.
- Pile several of the greens on top of each other and roll.
- Hold the rolled greens at the end and slice very fine. Move hand back away from knife as you proceed to finely chop the green. If you are short on time, use a food processor.
- Place greens in the mixing bowl.
- Add Olive oil or any other cold pressed oil.
- With your clean hands, massage the greens with the oil.
- Add all other ingredients and place in the refrigerator until serving time.

Ananse Ntontan

Carrot Sprout Salad

1 cup lentil sprouts
olive oil
cumin
turmeric
cayenne pepper
2 cups carrots, grated (using the grating disc of a food processor)
½ c coriander, chopped
lemon juice
¼ c green sprouts of your choice
¼ c soaked almond slices
dash of Bragg liquid amino

- Toss the lentil sprouts with the cumin, turmeric, cayenne pepper and a dash of olive oil and lemon juice until well-coated. You don't need much of the oil or lemon juice, just enough to help coat the sprouts with the seasonings.
- Put the lentil sprouts in a large bowl with the grated carrots and coriander.
- Toss everything with lemon juice and a touch of olive oil to taste.

Zucchini Salad

Dice 3 medium-sized zucchini
½ c red onion
1 large sliced organic tomato
1 ripe organic avocado
Add 2 tablespoons Veganaise
1 T spicy brown or Dijon mustard
2 pieces of soy bacon for garnish (optional)

- Cut and mix all ingredients, except avocado and vegan bacon.
- Let vegetables marinate for at least 15 before serving this tasty eye appealing dish.
- Add Avocado and garnish with veggie bacon and fresh parsely.
- Serve on a bed of sprouts, wrap in a green leaf or in a sprouted grain tortilla that has been warmed in a skillet.
- Bubbies organic dills might also be good in this salad.

Green Wraps

Use collard greens that you have cut away the stem to wrap up the contents. Use this method to reduce the amount of bread you are eating and to increase your green leaf intake. If you choose to eat the collard raw you might want to prepare a dipping sauce, or use a ready-made salad dressing or Veganaise.

The Collards can also be dipped in hot water for less than 10 seconds, this will soften them. The outer leaves of a cabbage can be used the same way. Eating green wraps will fill you up and not expand your body temple.

Ananse Ntontan

Tasty Red Cabbage Salad

Red Cabbage chopped thin and in bite-sized pieces
Spring onions
Tomatoes
Green olives or capers
Tahini sauce (sesame tahini. lemon juice, garlic powder)
If you don't have Tahini sauce, just use your favorite salad
dressing. Don't get stuck, be creative!

Chop, pour, let it sit for about 30 serve at room temperature.

'Light and sweet', add
1c Dried organic apricots
1c Pistachios
¼ cup organic dates (to sweeten)

Grind in food processor.

Coconut Bacon Chips

One bag of large coconut chips
Marinate in Tamari sauce and smoked paprika
Spread out on a flat baking pan and bake at 350 for 15-25
minutes turning when brown
Remove from oven and let cool before consuming.
Good as a salad topping
A very tasty bacon-like snack

Raw Egusi Soup
Chef Heru Harold Goodridge

¾ c pumpkin seeds
¾ c cashews
6 large tomatoes, chopped
1c soaked sundried tomatoes
1 small onion, chopped
2 habanero peppers, seeded and minced
2T of red palm oil
2c of finely cut spinach or any green leafy veg
1 t coarse salt - Celtic or Himalayan

Place pumpkin seeds in a blender and blend for 30-40 seconds or until mixture is a powdery paste. Place in a bowl.
Place cashews in a blender and blend for 30-40 seconds or until mixture is a powdery paste.
Transfer to the pumpkin seed mixture.
Place chopped tomatoes, sundried tomatoes, onions, red palm oil and pepper in a blender and blend for 30 seconds or until smooth.
Transfer mixture the bowl of pumpkins seeds and cashews.
Mix all ingredients.
Add spinach and sea salt and mix until well blended.

Ananse Ntontan

Avocado Dream Soup
Chef Elaine Rice-Fells

Eat immediately. Does not keep overnight or for later.

Meat of 1 ripe avocado (one of a few good fats)
3 T Nama Shoyu or Celtic sea salt to taste
¼ c fresh squeezed lime juice
¼ bunch fresh cilantro
¼ t ground cumin
3-4 cloves garlic
¾ c warm water
Place all ingredients in your blender and blend until desired smoothness.
Sprinkle on top any item that you think will taste good:
Diced red, yellow or orange bell pepper, chopped spring onions, cayenne pepper, paprika, chili powder, chopped celery
Serves 1-2

Avocado Wrap or Sandwich

When Avocado is soft to touch cut in half around seed
Take one half and cut into slivers and scoop out of shell,
cut only what you need leave rest in shell
Place on your flat sprouted grain tortilla or nori paper
or sprouted bread. Season with garlic powder or hing
and a natural salt
Add sprouts or lettuce or spinach
Tomatoes and vegan cheese (commercial or homemade - See Linda Carter recipe, page 22).
Add your dress and veg out!

Raw Sharp Cheese
Chef Linda Carter

1 T red wheat berries
1/2 pound pumpkin seeds
2 T miso paste
Juice of two limes
Pinch of Salt
Nutritional yeast to taste
Soak wheat berries in 2c water for two days or until you see fermentation
Strain the berries and save the water
Soak pumpkin seeds 4 hours, then rinse water off.
In a blender add pumpkin seeds- miso paste, fermented water, lime juice and salt.
Blend until creamy and smooth!

Spinach Spread
Chef Elaine Rice-Fells

1 Bunch spinach
½ c parsley
2 T raw almond butter
If you don't have almond butter I have used soaked almonds.
Squirt of Nama Shoyu
Olive or flax oil
Juice of 1 lemon
1 garlic clove minced
Blend all in the food processor.
Eat with crackers or alone.

Live Garlic Bread
Chef Elaine Rice-Fells

Yields 2 small 'loaves'

2 c almond pulp
1 c young coconut meat
1 c psyllium
½ c flax meal
3 t lemon juice
2 cloves crushed garlic
2 t garlic powder
3 soft dates
1 t salt

Blend the coconut meat, garlic and dates in a high-speed blender until smooth.
Grind that mixture with all remaining ingredients in a food processor until thoroughly combined.
Form into 2 loaves (1″ by 2″) wide.
Dehydrate on a mesh sheet for 14 hours at 115°F.
Remove from the dehydrator and cut into slices.
Stores in the refrigerator for up to 4 days

Eggplant Bacon
Chef Elaine Rice-Fells

1 or 2 large eggplant, thinly sliced, lengthwise
1 T Celtic sea salt
½ dried chipotle chili, soaked in ½ c water
½ c soaking water from chipotle chili
2 T grade B maple syrup
2 T extra-virgin Olive Oil
2 T tamari Sauce
2 T apple cider vinegar
1 t chili powder
½ t smoky paprika
½ t cumin

Toss eggplant and sea salt in a large bowl and let sit
1-2 hours.
Blend remaining ingredients in vita-mix and place in
medium-sized bowl.
Drain liquid from eggplant and add slices to bowl with
marinade.
Allow eggplant to marinate 30-45 minutes or longer.
Spread slices on dehydrator screens.
Dehydrate 24-30 hours at 110 degrees or longer until crisp.

NOT MEATS

Sun Power Nuggets
Chef Heru

2c sunflower seeds
½ c olive oil
1c finely chopped onion
1c finely chopped celery
1T curry
1 t rosemary
2 cloves garlic
1 teaspoon of salt
1 tablespoon No Salt Spike seasoning

Soak the sunflower seeds for two hours.
Drain the sunflower seeds.
Grind in food processor with garlic, olive oil, onions, celery until smooth.
Transfer the mixture to a bowl and add the remaining ingredients.
Place 2 tablespoons of the mixture on a dehydrator tray and shape into a round ball.
Dehydrate the nuggets at 110 for 4 hours.
You can also use the oven at the lowest temperature.

Ankh Life Meat
Chef Heru

Equipment needed - food processor

1 c walnuts
½ c sunflower seeds
½ c pumpkin seeds
½ c sun-dried tomatoes (or replace the sun dried tomatoes with red bell peppers)
1 c diced red bell peppers
1 c diced celery
½ c finely diced sweet onions
¼ c finely chopped parsley
1 T olive oil
1 T dried seasonings

Soak the walnuts, sunflowers, and pumpkin seeds in water for eight hours, drain the soaked seeds, and then rinse them in water. Drain them again.

Place the nuts and seeds into a food processor with an s-blade attachment and mix until finely grounded. Transfer the finely grounded nuts and seeds to a bowl.

Place the sun dried tomatoes, red bell peppers, olive oil in a food processor with an s-blade. Process until the mixture is thick and chunky. Transfer the mixture to the bowl with the finely grounded nuts and seeds. Add the diced celery, diced sweet onions, chopped parsley, and dried seasonings.

Mix until all ingredients are well blended.

ENTREES AND A LA CARTE

Vegan Tempeh BBQ sticks

One or two pounds per person
Purchase tempeh at Trader Joe's for best value
Cut in half lengthwise
Next chop into ¾-inch sticks

Season with:
Garlic powder
Dash of red pepper (more if children are not going to partake)
Himalayan salt
Cumin, optional

Squeeze lemon juice over sticks just enough to cover.
Let marinate for at least an hour.
A dash of Bragg's or tamari is great with this as well.
After marinating, pan-brown on one side before turning over.
Use coconut oil. Turn to other side.

When done, drizzle your favorite BBQ sauce and serve with broccoli and tomatoes.
They will love you!

Eggplant Fish

You can substitute eggplant in this recipe for tempeh.
I like both, I think eggplant has less calories.
Wash and peel egg plant, cut in half the cut into one/two inch half round.
Lay on a baking sheet and salt with a healthy salt.
Not much salt is needed, so don't be heavy handed.
After a few minutes pat with paper towel.
This will draw out bitterness.
Now your eggplant steaks are ready to be seasoned and dipped into milk and corn meal. Follow same directions as in tempeh fish recipe (below).
The eggplant should still be firm after cooking.

Tempeh Fish
Adapted from *Eat Like a Vegan* on Hulu

Cut Tempeh in half then cut it lengthwise , so it is thinner.
Cut all pieces on the diagonal so you end up with a triangle.
Season with:
Garlic powder
Kelp powder or Old Bay
Red pepper
Bragg, Tamari, Sea salt, or a good salt of choice

Squeeze lemon over pieces and massage gently.
Let sit for one hour.
Next dip in a bowl of Coconut milk
Then dip in some organic cornmeal, double dip if you like.
Place in your medium heated black skillet and brown
Place on paper towel after browning both sides.

Ananse Ntontan

Prepare some Veganaise for a tarter like sauce.
You can also use an organic low sug ketchup.
Serve with broccoli and a salad.

Veggie Patties

2 c soaked garbanzo beans for 24 hours
1 c quinoa or millet
3 grated carrots
garlic powder
cumin powder
ginger
thyme
diced red onions
chopped spinach
1T miso
2T nut butter
1 medium tomato diced
Diluted Bragg aminos to taste

Mix well and pan brown with cold-pressed grapeseed oil or organic cold pressed coconut oil. Make a sandwich with Ezekiel sprouted bread or tortilla. Weight conscious, then wrap in collard leaf, after you have removed the stem in the center, add your garnish and Veganaise and really enjoy.

Falafel

Don't have time to make the veggie patties, buy some Falafel mix from the organic market add water and grated veggies of your choice and take it to a medium warm skillet. Test one then put your mark on the rest of the batter with additional seasoning of your choice. Purchase the falafel mix in the bulk section of your Organic market. Check the salt content, some box mixes are very high in sodium.

Quinoa Tabuleh
Chef Elaine Rice-Fells

Prep Time after soaking, about an hour.

Equipment needed :
Food Processor or your choice of a chopper
Chef and Paring Knife (sharpened) or your favorite knife
Bowls, Rubber Spatulas and Cutting Board
Serves: 3-4

¼ c quinoa (1/8 Cup Red, 1/8 Cup white for color) sprouted
1/8 c dried burdock root (if fresh, chop fine, if dry soak for 6-8 hours)
1 bunch parsley
½ bunch cilantro chopped
½ c grape tomatoes quartered
½ c sundried tomatoes soaked for 2 hours, drained and chopped
½ large cucumber peeled and diced small (remove seeds)
1 T minced fresh ginger
¼ t ground cumin
2 cloves garlic minced

Ananse Ntontan

¼ c fresh-squeezed lemon juice
1 T minced habanera pepper (remove seeds for less heat)
OPTIONAL
2-3 T each of red and green onions chopped
¼ c black Moroccan olives pitted and cut in half
3 T nama shoyu or Celtic sea salt to taste OPTIONAL
¼ c extra-virgin olive oil (add more if desired)
½ t agave' nectar OPTIONAL

In a bowl, place quinoa with just enough water to cover.
Let soak overnight or 8 hours until tiny white sprouts
are visible.
Drain, rinse well and drain again.
Allow the burdock root to soak in water overnight or
8 hours as well.
Drain, rinse well and drain again.
Prepare all remaining ingredients as mentioned above
Add all ingredients with quinoa and burdock root in a large
bowl then mix thoroughly.
Serve immediately or allow to meld up to two hours
to savor all the flavors.
Serve as a side dish, on a bed of your favorite salad greens
or enjoy alone.

Tasty Green Beans

3-4 c of Organic Green beans
Wash and snap ends on beans, snap into bit size pieces
¼ c Onions
2T Miso broth or vegan chicken cube
2 cloves chopped Garlic or garlic powder
Grated carrots
Diluted Aminos

Cook green beans in seasoned vegetable broth at med/low
heat, as to not kill all the nutrients.
Cook for 20-30 minutes.
Beans should still have some texture and crunch, which
means you will benefit from the dish nutritionally- speaking
and you will not over eat.
Add grated carrots.

Quick Skillet Veggies

Start with onions and tomatoes
Add seasonings of choice: Garlic powder, Cumin,
Curry, Thyme, Oregano
Diluted Bragg aminos
Grapeseed oil

Sautee in skillet , add the other veggies according to firmness
of vegetable, the soft ones are cooked last.
Add ¼ cup filtered water, turn down heat and let the veggies
simmer. Serve with quinoa, basmati rice, millet
Or small grain brown rice.

Add veggies, diced zucchini, yellow squash, chopped kale, or
baby spinach.

Ananse Ntontan

Enchiladas

1 medium red onion, chopped fine
2 cloves garlic cloves, minced
12 ounces patty pan, zucchini, or yellow summer squash, diced (about 2 medium squash)
½ t ground cumin
1 t Ancho chile powder (or mild chili powder)
1/8 -1/4 t chipotle chile powder (or to taste)
1-½ c cooked black beans, well rinsed and drained
1 t of Bragg liquid aminos
1 T nutritional yeast
2 t lime juice
1 enchilada sauce/ seasoned tomato sauce and thicken with arrowroot
5-7 corn tortillas
chopped green onions, for serving

Sauté the onion in a medium-sized saucepan until it begins to soften.
Add the garlic and cook for another minute.
Stir in squash and cook, stirring, for about two minutes, until squash is just beginning to become tender.
Add the cumin, chile powders, black beans, and salt. Simmer for 5 minutes.
Remove from heat and stir in the nutritional yeast and lime juice.
Check seasoning and adjust to taste.
Preheat oven to 350.
Lightly spray one large rectangular baking dish or
4 individual baking dishes with olive oil.
Place a thin layer of enchilada sauce on the bottom of each dish, reserving most of it to go on top.
Place a tortilla in front of you and arrange about ¼ cup of

the bean mixture across the center.
Roll up and place seam-side down into the baking dish.
Repeat with remaining tortillas and beans.
Pour the remaining sauce over the top.
Bake for about 20 minutes, or until hot and bubbling.
Sprinkle with sliced green onions to serve.

Makes 6 servings

Vegan Cabbage Rolls
Chef Tomi Makajuola, The Vegan Nigerian

Ingredients
6 large cabbage leaves
handful chopped peanuts
For the peanut sauce:
1 tin chopped tomatoes
1 red bell pepper
2 or 3 small chillies (chopped)
2 small red onions (cut into rings)
1 garlic clove (finely chopped)
1 tbsp olive oil
1 tbsp peanut butter
salt to taste

Fill a large pot with lightly salted water and bring to a boil.
Add the large cabbage leaves and blanch for about 8-10 minutes to soften the leaves a little. Take out and allow to cool.
Then use a small knife to trim the thick part of the rind so that the leaf can fold easily.

Start to make the peanut sauce. Blend the chopped tomatoes with the red bell pepper and 2 chilis to form a slightly chunky sauce. Heat some olive oil in a large saucepan and sauté the chopped red onions and garlic for a minute or so, stirring constantly. Add the blended tomato/pepper sauce and some extra chopped chili if you want the extra spice. Turn the heat to medium. Allow to boil for 5 minutes before stirring in a tablespoon of peanut butter. Season with a bit of salt, turn the heat down, allow to simmer for another 10-15 minutes.

For the filling
1 small sweet potato (cooked, flesh only)
1 cup cooked beans
½ tsp curry powder
1 tsp dried thyme
Mash all the filling ingredients together in a large bowl.

To assemble the cabbage roll, place about a table-spoon of the filling into the center of the leaf, fold one side over, roll the cabbage into a parcel and tuck in the sides on each end to secure. Repeat the process with the rest of the leaves and filling. Arrange the cabbage rolls into a rectangular baking dish, seam side facing down.

Spoon the red peanut sauce evenly over the top.
Bake in a pre-heated oven for 15-20 minutes until piping hot.
Serve with some chopped peanuts sprinkled over the top!

Serves 2-3

Spinach and Pine Nuts
Chef Sheeba Ema-Nuru

- 2½ pounds spinach
- 2 to 3 tablespoons olive oil
- 2 small yellow onions or 6 green onions, minced
- 4 tablespoons raisins, soaked in water and drained
- 4 tablespoons pine nuts raw
- pinch of sea salt or dash of diluted Bragg liquid aminos

Rinse the spinach well and remove the stems.
Place in a large sauté pan with only the rinsing water clinging to the leaves.
Cook over medium heat, turning as needed until wilted, just a few minutes.
Drain well and set aside.
Add the olive oil to the now-empty pan and place over medium heat.
Add the onions and sauté until tender, about 8 minutes.
Add the spinach, raisins, and pine nuts and sauté briefly to warm through.
Season and enjoy.

Ananse Ntontan

Cooked Collard Greens

2 bunches small leaf collard greens
¼ c olive oil or other cold pressed oil

Wash and remove some of the stem. Cut in thin strips.
Massage olive oil into your greens.
1 onion
1 tomato
garlic powder
onion powder
cumin powder
bay leaf
Bragg liquid aminos
1/2cup filtered water

Lightly saute your seasoning veggies, add water, stir.
Add the prepared collard greens to the pot, mix well, close
the lid and let steam for about 15 minutes at medium low
heat , until tender, don't cook all the life/enzymes out of
them.

Sweet Potatoes

Bake or boil until tender.
Cut open add some coconut oil instead of butter.
Sprinkle on some cinnamon and enjoy!
Serve with Tempeh and greens cooked or raw!

Vegetarian Stuffed Cheese Shells
Chef Kunti Hawkins

Large jumbo whole grain pasta shells
Frozen spinach
Organic or vegan Parmesan cheese
Organic or vegan Mozzarella cheese
Organic or vegan Ricotta cheese
Crushed tomatoes about 2 cans
Hing
Basil fresh
Italian seasonings
Oregano
Asafetida
Old Bay
Salt
Maple syrup to taste

Boil water add oil to water cook pasta
Drain water and wash with cold water
Set aside

In a separate pot, heat oil slightly add hing
Then add crushed tomatoes and cook on medium heat
Add other all the other ingredients: oregano, old bay, Italian
seasons and maple syrup and salt, cook at med to low heat.
Cook frozen spinach in separate pot and drain.
Squeeze out excess water from spinach.
In a bowl add cheeses and save some mozzarella for topping.
Add spinach
Old bay
Add basil
Add Italian seasoning
Hing

Ananse Ntontan

Salt to taste
Mix all well
Stuff mixture into cooked pasta shells
Line in a baking pan, salt
Top with sauce and garnish with mozzarella.
Bake for 30-45 minutes for 350 until nice and golden

Veggie Deluxe Pizza
Chef Dr. Akua Gray

½ red bell pepper
½ yellow bell pepper
½ green bell pepper
½ red onion
½ yellow onion
2 stalks of green onion
3 cloves of garlic
1 cup broccoli
¼ cup of fresh parsley

Heat oven to 200°. Prepare pizza crust of choice, a vegan variety, with marinara sauce and set aside. Chop green onions and slice all other vegetables into very thin long slices. Sautee lightly with a little olive oil and top waiting pizza crust. Heat in oven for 10 – 15 minutes or until crust is warmed. Slice and serve.

Vegan Chili

Soak red beans, mung bean and black beans overnight
If you have time let sprout for a couple of days
Season a slow cooker with coconut oil
Add red pepper, garlic powder and hing and a quality
salt of your choice.
Add beans and stir so all the spices are coving the beans.
Cook like this for 5-10 minutes.
Then add water to cook beans.
Slow cook overnight on low.
When the beans are soft add tomato sauce, celery,
a bay leaf and chopped carrots.
When veggies are tender but not overcooked, add some
broccoli florets and stir well.
When broccoli is tender, but not soft serve your chili.
Serve with a small grain brown rice and a green salad.

TASTY TREATS

Popcorn Balls

Dried dates moistened with coconut water, or any liquid
desired, gently, do not soak. Grind in food processor, consistency should be slightly chunky. Place in mixing bowl
Organic non-gmo popcorn, popped - gently grind in food
processor, should have some texture when finished.
Do not over grind.
Sesame seeds whole or ground in coffee grinder
Orange peel or Youngliving essential oil of Orange, stick tooth
pick in jar and then into food. Straight from bottle may spoil
the dish. (optional)

Mix all ingredients and form into tasty balls. Refrigerate until
serving time. The kids and your guests will love them!

Ananse Ntontan

Chocolate Pudding

2 medium/large avocados
1 c water
¼ c cacao powder or more to taste
(depends on the size of the avocados)
¼ c of agave nectar
1 t vanilla extract

Combine all ingredients in a food processor and puree until smooth, adding a little more water if needed. More water will give you a thinner pudding.
Serves 4

Carob or Raw Cacao/Peppermint Brownie

1 c carob or Cacao (Carob is a raw food)
2 c almond meal or cashew meal
Add organic apple juice to moisten batter,
should still be thick
Add Vanilla flavoring, cinnamon and a pinch of nutmeg
Stick a toothpick into a Young Living bottle of peppermint oil,
then place the tooth pick in your batter, repeat for more
flavor, then remove.
Add Stevia for sweetness or natural sweeteners
½ c soaked flax seed to bind
Cinnamon
Add chopped soaked walnuts
Stir and mix into a thick consistency.
Place in a pan, loaf or cake pan, place in freezer for a couple
of hours to harden, then slice as needed.
Serve at room temperature
Garnish with raspberries.

Quick & Easy, Raw, Key Lime Pudding
Chef Elaine Rice-Fells

- 1 ripe avocado (peeled & pitted)
- 1 ripe banana (peeled)
- 1 tablespoon raw coconut oil
- Juice from ½ a lemon
- Juice from ½ a lime

Place all ingredients in a food processor and process until smooth.

For Crust: In a food processor, process 2 cups of almonds or nuts of your choice along with 4-6 dates. Press into a spring-form pan or Pyrex then pour in pie mixture and allow to chill for a few hours then serve.
ENJOY!

Raw Peach Pudding
Chef Dr. Akua Gray

4 ripe peaches with skins
½ c almond meal
1 teaspoon vanilla optional

Blend in food processor to desired texture. If not sweet enough for you use stevia or a ripe banana. Wonderful breakfast item!

Ananse Ntontan

Fruity Chia Seed Pudding
Chef Sheeba Ema-Nuru

This recipe is a good protein-packed snack that can keep in the fridge until you need it and is really perfect for people on the go!

1c raspberries (or whichever berry is your favorite)
½ c coconut meat
1½ c coconut water
1/3 c agave or honey
¼ t sea salt
3/4 c white chia seeds

Blend all the ingredients (except for the chia seeds)
until smooth.
Pour mixture into a serving bowl.
Pour the chia seeds into the berry mixture,
stirring constantly.
Place bowl in refrigerator to set for at least 30 minutes.
If the consistency is too thick for you, add more
coconut water.
If it's not thick enough, add more chia seeds.
Enjoy!

Nsoromma

Children of the Stars

TIPS FOR MAINTAINING YOUR VEGAN LIFESTYLE

Transitioning can be a challenge and sometimes your new vegan support group won't be enough to get you through. Here are some lists and tips to help you maintain a plant based consciousness in your busy lifestyles.

WHEN TIME IS AN ISSUE

1. Fruit
2. Dried fruits
3. Raw nuts or seeds
4. Organic baked chips
5. Seaweed Nori sheets
6. Baked organic crackers
7. 100% Juice organic diluted with alkaline water
8. Organic bag of salad or spinach, make a salad
9. Plantain Chips baked
10. Rice crackers
11. Organic hummus w/o canola oil
12. Burrito with sprouted grains, salad, hummus, olives and a dressing
13. Bake or boil a sweet potato or yam
14. African yams, do not overcook very nutritious
15. Sauté some frozen veggies with tomatoes and onions and seasoning, top with baby spinach
16. Non soy veggie meat product - burger, link etc.

Make a sandwich with sprouted grain bread
17. Make a smoothie; load it up with protein powder, moringa, spirulina etc. Use frozen berries, apples, and green leafy veggies
18. Sauté a plantain in a little oil, season it to match your mood, sweet or savory.
19. Buy an organic pizza crust, add vegan cheese or make one from our recipe section, load up with veggies and olives and dried tomatoes.
20. Buy some sprouts and vegenaise. This will give you immediate energy. Place in nori seaweed paper or eat as a salad. Season lightly with spike.
21. Soak some lentils for about an hour, cook with seasoning and oil. Add other veggies like carrots and tomatoes, red onion and you have a nice soup in 2 hours.
22. Make a raw soup. Purchase chopped butternut squash, boil some water, add your seasonings and place in vita-mixer until soup. Add a little coconut oil. You can do this with any vegetable, hot water, and your high powered blender.
23. Ruben Sandwich gone veg sandwich, toasted sprouted bread, vegenaise, sauerkraut, tomato, avocado and vegan cheese .
24. A bowl of strawberries or any fruit
25. Strawberries, coconut yogurt, granola
26. Organic popcorn
27. Crack some coconuts and drink the water, make milk with the rest.
28. BLT on sprouted grains with tempeh bacon, tomato, sprouts, vegenaise and dried tomatoes
29. Bananas and peanut butter or any organic nut butter, pricey, (but so easy to make) on sprouted bread.
30. Buy some artichokes hearts in the jar or olive spread, make a dip or sandwich or top your salad

31. Buy some collards, cut the stem out and use as a roll with whatever you choose. Can be dipped in some hot water before adding ingredients to soften.
32. Buy some east Indian food in the cooking bags, boil and chop!
33. Make soup using miso and add other veggies and seasonings.
34. Some gari and top with veggies. Gari is dried cassava, purchase in the Afrikan Market.
35. Make some hot water cornbread and eat with your salad or sautéed veggies. Ingredients: Organic corn meal, baking soda, coconut oils, dash of Himalayan salt, hot water. Batter should be thick, not too much water. Experiment: Make into patties and pan fry. Feel free to load up with diced veggies once you get the hang of it.

Eating Vegan on the Cheap

Many complain that it is expensive to eat healthy. To a degree this is true. There are ways to work around it. This list was created to help you with your Healing Room/kitchen economics.

1. Gardening can take many different aspects, depending on where you live. Get your hands soil-y.
   a. Plant a garden in the ground
   b. Plant a container garden
   c. Plant an indoor or outdoor herb garden
   d. Plant in a child's rubber swimming pool
   e. Learn how to sprout and sprout in your (kitchen) in the soil.
   f. Learn to dehydrate and store foods
   g. Buy a dehydrator or use the oven at the lowest temperature
   h. Learn how to can foods in mason jars

      i.   Planting from seed is most economical

      j.   Buy a small green house so you can grow something in the winter.

2. Shop at the farmer's market, or go to the farm.
3. Buy uncertified organic, from a trusted farmer. Some farmers do not get certified because it is rather costly- but they do not use any herbicides or pesti cides. If you know your farmer well, this is a perfectly fine solution.
4. Make your own vegan dairy products, nut milks, cheeses, etc.
5. Use coupons.
6. Visit u-pick farms for fruits and berries, then preserve them by canning or freezing.
7. Shop with a keen eye for trusted brands in low cost stores like Big Lots for items you can use and look for organic items.
8. Eat foods in season.
9. Eating high-Live will cut your need for more and more food. I would suggest at least 50/50 if you are not battling disease. If you are sick then the more live foods the better, along with juicing.
10. The more you hang out in the kitchen the more you are going to eat. (The kitchen is not a good place for your office.)
11. Drink more water. Sometimes we think we are hungry when really the body needs good clean alkaline water.
12. Ask for what you need for your birthday, anniversary Kwanzaa etc.
13. Shopping online you can find some great deals!
14. Whole Foods can overwhelm you with all the beautiful things to buy. Take a list and stick to it.
15. Each chain store has a newspaper of sales, study it

before you begin. Get on the store's mailing list for specials.

16. Got extra money and storage? Buy in bulk when you can.

17. Team up with friends, you do the cooking they buy the groceries, or pay you to cook. If the latter, you may need a food handlers license.

18. Fresh is best, but sometimes homey gotta buy frozen, make sure it is organic.

19. If you shop once every seven days, then make a mental note not to consume for example all the olives before your day 6 or 7.

20. See what you have on hand as a blessing and create with it!

21. Know that more is coming and give thanks!

22. Walk fast away from sections in the store that call you but aren't good for you. The bakery section, cheese etc.

23. When you can, buy local and unpackaged.

24. Sometimes if I don't have the cash, I will purchase the conventional item...but not all the time, as this would compromise my health.

25. Learn to make delicious soaked beans and grains. Learn to sprout them. This will save a ton of money and boost your health and beauty index!

26. Before you get in line at the store take out the extra stuff you don't need due to processing sugar, salt content or emotional buying. Ok, keep just one item!

27. Buy these items once then sprout them in water then plant. Carrots, basil, bok choi romaine lettuce, garlic, scallions and celery.
    Check out www.positivegardening.com for more info.

Traveling While Vegan

Because you don't want to fail, you must plan before you get in the wind, on the road or in the waters. Here are some suggestions that will help you to be a successful vegan while moving around your world.

1. Be gentle on yourself, you may not be able to keep up your vegan discipline as well on the road as when at home.
2. Pack a stick blender for smoothies and soups.
3. Pack a portable toaster to warm up foods, because micro-waves are not good for you or your food.
4. Pack a small citrus juicer.
5. Make or buy some crackers.
6. Make or buy some hummus.
7. Purchase some roasted seaweed.
8. Pack a cooler and put your perishables inside. Make sure it has the ice inserts.
9. Pack coconut water.
10. Make or purchase trail mix, healthy ones.
11. Water and juice is a must.
12. Miso instant soup is a winner!
13. Pack some veggies, add to soups, wraps and use for main course.
14. Always book a room with a kitchenette that is stocked with utensils and a blender.
15. If you can't a take a cooler purchase an insulated backpack for food storage.
16. Make several dishes ahead of time and freeze for travel.
17. Do your homework before you get on the road - know spots where you can eat, shop organic or fresh, know where the health food stores are located. Ask about Nubian-owned and Seven Day Adventist restaurants

and locations.

18. If the location does not have a health food store ask where is the people's market. Take a local with you if you don't speak the language.

19. Call the hotel ahead of time and let them know you will be in the house and you are a vegan. Ask them to accommodate you.

20. Talk with the Chef. Then don't forget to praise them profusely when they do you right! Ok tip.

21. If the hotel has a store, check with the manager, order what you want from the market. I always do this in Mexico.

22. Speaking of Mexico, I sometimes find myself a vegetarian and not a vegan when traveling. I don't trip on this, but I will do a cleanse as soon as I come home. I chalk it up to it's a vacation. But don't go off the deep end.

23. Take kitchen supplies with you like small bottles of oil, spices, Bragg's etc. Make sure you can get through customs if you are out the country. Research the rules on food. If you are a baller, then skip these frugal suggestions. But they will save someone time and energy of run around getting supplies in a place that is relatively unknown.

24. Are you a Baller? hire a vegan chef!

25. Refresh your supplies for the trip home.

26. Research the airports for hip vegan eat spots. San Francisco's airport has really great places to eat.

27. In a crunch I will order juice, salad and a baked potato, ok, ok sometimes fries.

28. Gari a dried granulated product, can be purchase in an African international store, it is dried cassava which is in the yam family. Just add water to it and you have a good carb. Also it is great seasoned. Eat with your

soups or stews.

29. The item snacks should be divided up for travel, on location, and items that you will consume on the return trip.

30. Pack your Young Living Power Meal to add to your juice in the morning. Order from me, details in back of book. You could also order their vita greens for a multi green, lavender, or citronella essential oil for mosquito repellent.

31. I pack some of my supplements and take enough for the entire trip. In addition to supplements I will take Thieves Oil, and lemongrass. Thieves Oil helps to support your immune system and lemongrass is good to deal with any little parasites. Stress Away, as travel can be nerve racking. Travel size of Ningxia Red, which is a goji berry tonic. I drink it when others are having wine, and as a daily tonic. (www.Youngliving.com, use my number again 868573). They also have lots of healthy snacks that you can pack and go! Don't forget Ningxia Nitro for cognitive fitness. My new fav!

32. Depending on where you are going, consider packing charcoal tablets for digestive issues. Do your research.

33. Pack a wholistic natural emergency kit.

34. Pack some herbal teas.

35. I like ground, marinated sunflower seeds mixed with salsa, a good road snack.

36. Leave a bottle of water next to the sink where you brush your teeth in countries where the water is not potable.

37. I pack my own natural bath and body products, purchased from Youngliving.com.

38. While on the plane, I will use the Thieves' products to support my system against germs and not to mention recycled air. I use the essential oil on my person or I will put some on a cotton ball and place it in the air

School Lunches

The watoto (children) should be making this journey with you, in the long run you will simplify your life and stay the course if everybody in the family is on point. Children need to go to school with a plant based diet. Of course you could load them up with fake meat products which are processed and mostly soy, to send them off to school. That would be easy, but easy is not always the most enlightened path. Re-read the section on soy products if you have forgotten why we do not eat an abundance of soy products. You will want to help your child with a script when kids start the teasing. Give him words he can use. Like "to each to his own, my parents know what's best for me. At least I am eating real food." It has been a while since I had to make the mini-me a lunch for school, but here we go...

1. Purchase some baggies and a lunch box with different size containers to fill with your mostly homemade food.
2. Ask the child what they would like to have in the lunch. Lunch at a table full of kids collects lots of attention both supportive an unsupportive. That yummy peanut butter soup you made last night, just might make your child the butt of lots of jokes. Until they are strong enough and old enough to handle the critics I would choose foods that allow them to fit in.
3. Peanut butter on sprouted toast is always a winner. Drizzle w maple syrup or not, organic grapes, apple slices some crackers in a baggie and it's on!
4. The same lunch as above using a different nut butter. If it's too expensive, learn to make your own at home. Almond, cashew and sunflower seed butter are all good ones.

5. Use a cookie cutter on the sandwich to give it a theme and make it more desirable.
6. Peanut butter and bananas on sprouted grain bread.
7. (I like this one, you may not!) Peanut butter with dill pickle slices on hot toast.
8. Vegan spaghetti and meat balls, sprouted toast and veggie sticks.
9. Wraps are great for the lunch box. Sprouted tortilla wrap filled with veggies your child actually likes. Zucchini, carrots and tomatoes is a tasty choice.
10. Veggie burger on sprouted bread, Veganaise or dijon mustard, pickles, romaine lettuce and some sprouts is a winner.
11. Tacos made from organic corn filled with black beans, tomatoes, sprouts and Daiya or homemade cheese is a hip choice for lunch. Add some fruit and juice in a box and bam!
12. Bean soup with some homemade corn bread, veggie sticks and salad dressing and some water or juice and you are in!
13. Smoothies are a great addition to the lunch box. In the beginning make sure they are red with strawberries or cranberries and an apple, sneak in some sprouts, not too much. Add some youngliving power meal for a non-soy protein powder.
14. Make a vegetarian pizza and send it to school on pizza day. In a pinch- use an organic one you purchased.
15. I love hummus for lunches, use on a wrap with pickles, tomatoes and lettuce or sprouts. Send in lunch as a dip with veggie sticks.
16. Trail mixes are a great snack to have.
17. Coconut water is really nice in the hot seasons, as well as cool herb teas sweetened with stevia.
18. A nut milk shake is nice addition.

19. Carob because it looks like chocolate is a great addition. Make your own brownies with or raw treats. I really like granola bars but these days very high in sug sug /sugar. Shop around to find a good one.
20. Fruit salads are nice!
21. Cookies with healthy ingredients
22. Later when the child can navigate the nay sayers, you can send leftovers from the night before's dinner. Only if they actually like it.
23. There is a product called Field Roast, you can slice this and send to school as a sandwich. The kids will think he/she is eating meat. It is a gluten product. Seitan is another one. Not good if the child has any digestive issues, emotional issues or overweight.
24. Make a lunch date with the Watoto, sit in the cafeteria with your beloved and eat what they eat. This will give you a real perspective on what goes on in the lunch room.
25. Don't go berserk when they throw away your food or trade it for something less healthy and more appealing to their childish awareness. It happens, they are children. Just talk with them until you are blue in the face or until they grow up. Do experiments with them - soda pop and their teeth is a fun one. Place an old tooth in a jar of soda like coke or pepsi, return in a week and they will see with their own eyes why you don't give them this sugary chemical drink masquerading as food. They will know why they should not trade their good food for trash food at school. Teach them about eating and making good choices.
26. Then pray for them and leave them be! Don't get anal about this. Children learn differently than adults and

our expectations should be different. Just make sure the bulk of their food is homemade and plant based. I think it is easier when you start them out as infants on a plant based regime.

27. If you are a baller, go to whole foods and buy from the food court, make sure they like it, pack it up and send them off to school. I see frozen smoothies in the freezer department and wholesome Lunchables in the refrigerator section. This is ok once in a while.

28. Vegetarians, look in the frozen food section for real food you can send to school. Don't microwave!

29. I like some box items that are Indian, that can be boiled and served. Talk to cafeteria staff about doing this for your child.

30. Also talk with cafeteria staff about other ways they can accommodate your plant eater.

31. Join up with other parents and push your desires for more veggies that are not full of salt, sugar, chemicals and overcooked. a smoothie and/or salad bar would be a winner! All children would benefit from real food at lunch and breakfast. The PTA might want to head up a program for better lunches. Some schools have salad bars.

32. Stay away from traditional school lunches, they are generally bad news in most public schools. Go online and read the menu and the ingredients.

33. Ask the school counselor if she has an eating healthy support group, or if he/she is open to starting one.

34. Support your mini-me with books and learning opportunities on-line and off. The counselor should be able to support you if teasing becomes unmanageable.

35. Think ahead when it comes to school parties, holidays, the watoto are usually loaded down with junk

in public schools.

36. Think plantain chips and organic popcorn, apple sauce, coconut yogurt. Go to the bulk section of your health store to find treats for their lunch.

37. Don't forget fresh fruits. Always buy fruits with seeds. Seedless fruits could lead to infertility. Seedless humans?

Once you have read this document thoroughly, you are ready to start your journey to eating with mother nature, the goddess of health, vitality and longevity. She loves you and will treat you right.

A luta continua, the struggle continues and what you eat is definitely part of the NUBIAN struggle. We are ill with diabetes, obesity, high blood pressure, kidney disease, prostate, heart disease, cancers, and high infant mortality rates. We must liberate ourselves from improper diet and lifestyles. My prayer is that you will use this information to support your quest for better health. My prayer is that you use this booklet to help others, my prayer is that you will be guided to make some positive changes in your life to be an example for others to look up to. My hope is that you will become the nurturer in your family, circle of friends or community. The person who is okay with getting in the healing laboratory and hooking up healthy meals. The one who shuns the fast food joints that serve up plastic in your breads, silicone-like substances in the chicken and a host of other chemicals in products that should not be called food but edible chemicals.

'Each one-teach one' is a philosophy in our community that has always inspired others to move forward. Teach what you have learned and what you experience as a result of these practices.

Turning to a plant based diet in societies where animal slaughter is extensive is not easy. Take your time, be easy on yourself, but be persistent in your goals. Most of all plan every day before the sun rises, or plan to fail for that day. if you pray, affirm that you will receive guidance and support. Give thanks in advance.

Changing your diet will create space for better health and a higher frequency. Many teachers believe we are intentionally being numbed to dumb. Dumbed down by tv, movies, music, fluoride, chem-trails and of course chemical laden foods or chemical masquerading as food. This is but one way to keep yourself light and in light. Eat the plants, they are full of bright sun light.

This is one way for you to take control of your destiny. Take your stand, be natural, be healthy, be free from the corporate agenda of consumerism and disease. Wake up so you can awaken your family and friends, not by preaching to them but setting the example of health and vitality. Be your family's resource center. Stay on top of the information on foods and natural healing. Who knows? You may find a great enjoyment in learning and sharing info and create a new hobby/expertise or even a career, all the while gaining great positive karma from your service.

The sacred ancestors, angels and beings of light, will thank you. The earth will praise your name, as some of the animals who perhaps avoid slaughter. All things work together for the good. That's whats up with *Red, Black, Green and Vegan.*

"If we human beings are children of nature, then it is to nature we must look for our health, welfare, and survival."

Alvenia M. Fulton, Vegetarianism: Fact or Myth?
Eating to Live (Chicago: B.C.A. Publishing, 1978), II.

Bibliography

AfriKa, Llaila O. *African Holistic Health*

Campbell, T. Colin. *The China Study*

Fulton, Alvenia, ND, PHD, *Vegetarianism Fact or Myth*

Gregory, Dick. *Natural Diet for Folks Who Eat*

Kondo, Baba Zak A. *The Black Guide to Vegetarianism*, 1996. Nubian Press

Phahupada, A.C. Bhaktivedana Swami. 1983 Bhaktivedanta Books

Queen Afua, *Heal Thy Self*

The Higher Taste: A guide to Gourmet Vegetarian Cooking and a Karma-Free Diet, Based on The teachings of His Divine Grace

http://www.vrg.org/nutrition/

http://nutritionstudies.org/

AUTHOR INFORMATION
Zatiti Ema MA, CD, LMT, Certified Wholistic Healer

Living Foods Certification, Institute of Natural Health,
NADA-Certified
Global Sacred Woman/Queen Afua
Associate Teacher of Mantak Chia QiGong, ICTC Doula,LMT

CEO/Founder of The Healing Tree Detox Day Spa
The Healing Tree Detox Day Spa

Services:
Spa Days for men and women, single or group
Health Consultations, including foods, vitamins, aromatherapy and herbals

Detox Spa Services:
Infrared sauna
Aqua Chi
Steam sauna
Lady steam
Clay treatments
Color Treatments

Massage therapy:
Mobile or office
Swedish, Deep Tissue, Tui Na, Thai Yoga Massage,
Elder massage, sports massage, Reflexology,
Reiki and crystal treatments

Vegetarian/Vegan/Living Raw Foods support
Classes and Personal Chef Services
Doula Services

PRODUCTS

www.zatiti.juiceplus.com

Handmade all natural Soap and Bee's Wax Candles

Young Living Therapeutic Essential Oils,
Source for Natural Vitamins and Supplements
Call them the first time you order 1-800-371-3515
www.youngliving.com / **Use 868573**

Supplements/ vitimins
Emersonecologics.com
Use ht7971

Nubian-owned Health Establishments

Senbeb Natural Health Food Store and Café
Vegan/Raw Café & Catering
6224 3rd Street N.W.
Washington, D.C. 20011

Evolve
341 Cedar St N.W.
Takoma Park, MD 20012

Khepera Raw Food and Juice Bar
402 H Street N.E.
Washington D.C.
www.mojojuiceclub.com
Mojojuice@yahoogroups.com
zatiti.juiceplus.com

Secrets of Nature
3923 S. Capitol Street SW
Washington, DC

The Woodlands Vegan Bistro
2928 Georgia Ave NW
Washington, DC 20001

The Land of Kush
840 N. Eutaw St
Baltimore, MD

Brown's Health Food Market
5718 Silver Hill Road
District Heights, MD 20747

Veggie Delights Catering
DC/MD
240-286-3765

Vegan Flava Café Mobile
Raleigh/Durham,NC
Vegan Lover Catering
Chapel Hill, Raleigh, Durham

Soul Vegetarian
Tallahassee,Fl
Soul Vegetarian and Soul Vegetarian II
Atlanta, GA

The Original Soul Vegetarian
Chicago, IL

Tasilli's Raw Reality
1059 Ralph David Abernathy Blvd
Atlanta, GA 30310

Lovin it Live
2796 East Point Street
East Point,GA 30344

Two Vegan Sistas
Memphis, Tenn.

MAMA Atiola
Philadelphia, PA

E-LifeonWheel's 100% VeganFoodTruck
20th&L St NW DC

Everlasting Life
9185 Central Ave
Capitol Heights, Maryland
http://www.everlastinglife.net/

Non Nubian-owned Health Establishments

Arnold's Way
319 W Main Street
Store #4 Rear
Lansdale, PA 19446
215-316-0116

Bethesda Co-op
6500 Seven locks Rd., Cabin John, MD
301-320-2530

Glut Food Co-op
4005 34 St., Mt. Rainier, MD
301-779-1978
www.Glut.org

Online Resources

Nubian moderated:

Rawsoul@yahoogroups.com
Rawsoul-Rainbow colors facebook
Blacksgoingvegan.com
Vegansofcolor.wordpress.com
foodforthesoul.opare.net
bvsga.org
bvsdc.org
blackveggievegans/facebook.comhttp:
//www.drsebiscellfood.com/pages/nutritional-guide

Non Nubian
PETA.org
Animal right and vegetarianism

PCRM.org
Physicians Committee for Responsible Medicine

VegCooking.com
VegRecipes.org
Vegdc.com
Tryveg.com
  · Cok.net
  · www.veganrecipes.com
  · www.vegancooking.com
  · www.veganchef.com
  · www.ivu.org/recipes/
  · www.compassionatecooks.com
  · www.vegcooking.com

VIDEOS AND MOVIES*

Organic Life
Vegucated
Veggie Tales
Men Live on Plants Not Meat
Food Fight
Two Angry Moms
Genetically Modified Food
The Future of food
Super Size Me
Chow Down
Fat Head

Most of these can be viewed for free on Hulu. Search YouTube for more using vegetarian, vegan, living foods, sustainable living, organic and cruelty to animals in your search.

GARDENING

www. positivegardening.com

BOOKS

Afrika, Llaila O. *African Holistic Health*

Afua, Queen.
 Circles of Wellness: A Guide to Planting, Cultivating and Harvesting Wellness
 Heal Thyself for Health and Longevity

Amen, Ra Un Nefer. *Ausar Auset Nutrition Handbook*

Anu, Khepra. *Paradise Health: A festing and Fasting Guide to Optimal Health through Detoxification*